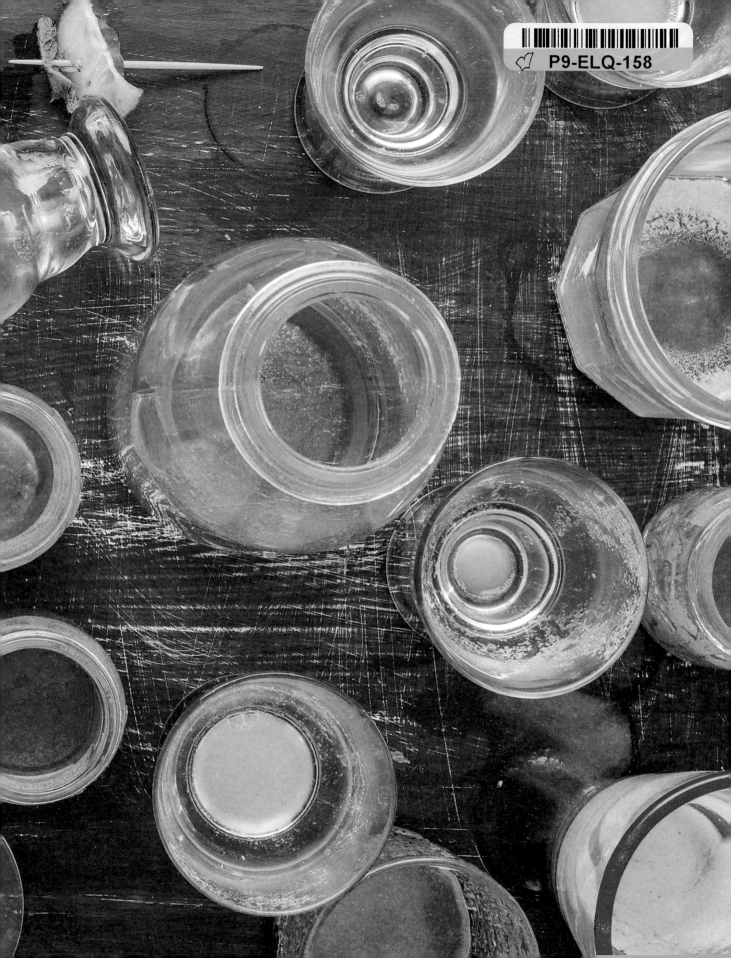

CLEAN & GREEN

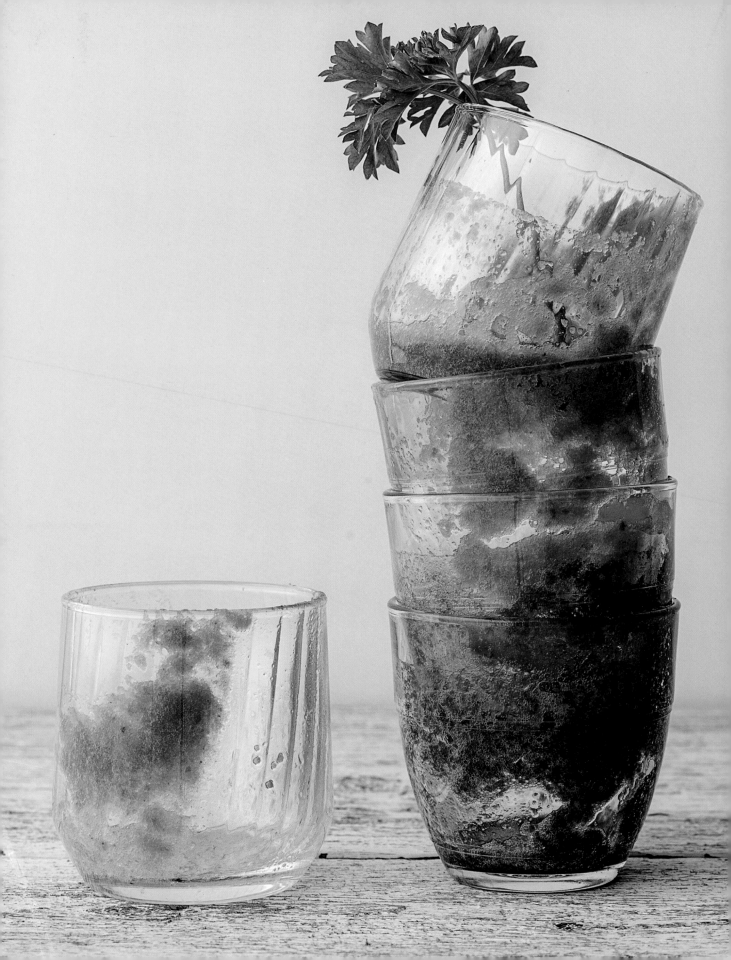

CLEAN & GREEN

LOVE FOOD™

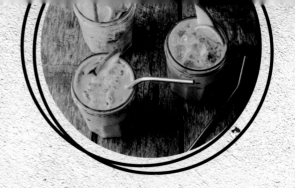

This edition published by Parragon Books Ltd in 2015
and distributed by

Parragon Inc.
440 Park Avenue South, 13th Floor
New York, NY 10016
www.parragon.com/lovefood

LOVE FOOD is an imprint of Parragon Books Ltd

ISBN 978-1-4723-8937-4

Printed in China

Project managed by Andrea O'Connor
New recipes by Mima Sinclair
Designed by Beth Kalynka
New photography by Max and Liz Haarala Hamilton
Introduction and additional text by Judith Wills
Production by Joe Xavier

Notes for the Reader
This book uses standard kitchen measuring spoons and cups. All spoon and cup
measurements are level unless otherwise indicated. Unless otherwise stated, milk
is assumed to be whole, eggs are large, individual vegetables are medium, and
pepper is freshly ground black pepper. Unless otherwise stated, all root vegetables
should be peeled prior to using. Garnishes, decorations, and serving suggestions
are all optional and not necessarily included in the recipe ingredients or method.

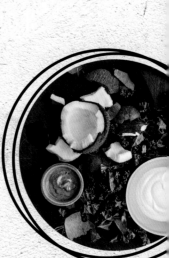

While the author has made all reasonable efforts to ensure that the information
contained in this book is accurate and up to date at the time of publication, anyone
reading this book should note the following important points:

Medical and pharmaceutical knowledge is constantly changing and the author and
the publisher cannot and do not guarantee the accuracy or appropriateness of the
contents of this book.

In any event, this book is not intended to be, and should not be relied upon, as a
substitute for appropriate, tailored professional advice. Both the author and the
publisher strongly recommend that a physician or other healthcare professional is
consulted before embarking on major dietary changes.

For the reasons set out above, and to the fullest extent permitted by law, the
author and publisher: (i) cannot and do not accept any legal duty of care or
responsibility in relation to the accuracy or appropriateness of the contents of this
book, even where expressed as "advice" or using other words to this effect; and
(ii) disclaim any liability, loss, damage, or risk that may be claimed or incurred as a
consequence—directly or indirectly—of the use and/or application of any of the
contents of this book.

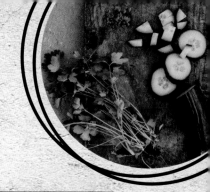
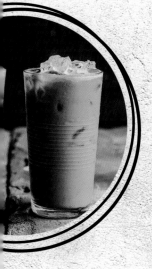

CONTENTS

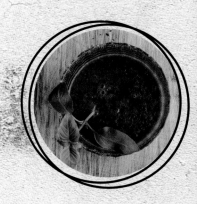
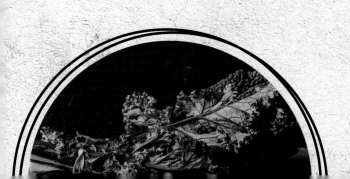

WHY GOING GREEN IS GOOD FOR YOUR HEALTH

GREEN JUICING IS NO LONGER THE PRESERVE OF MOVIE STARS, SUPERMODELS, AND VEGANS. EVERYONE'S GONE MAD FOR IT, AND NO WONDER. IF YOU WANT TO LOOK AFTER YOUR HEALTH, WELL-BEING, WEIGHT, AND APPEARANCE, THERE IS SURELY NO EASIER WAY TO DO IT THAN BY INCORPORATING JUICING INTO YOUR DIET.

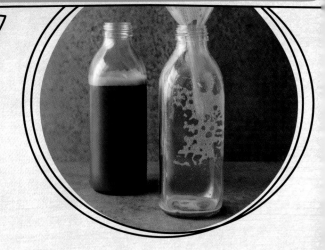

SO, WHO IS IT IDEAL FOR?

Virtually everyone can benefit from including green juices, smoothies, shots, and soups in their diet. They're easy, quick to make, and great for people short on time. They're portable, too—so make and take to the office—and versatile, with sweet, sour, savory, and spicy notes.

WHY IS IT SO HEALTHY?

With ingredients such as raw vegetables and fruit as well as health-boosting micro-ingredients, herbs, and spices, clean and green recipes literally are a health boost in a glass—or bowl. If you juice regularly, you'll be getting all the vitamins and minerals you need, a high level of antioxidants, and various types of dietary fiber.

HOW TO BUY THE FRESHEST INGREDIENTS

Always buy the best-quality, freshest products you can find—they contain more nutrients and flavor. Organic produce should be first choice where possible. Try buying at a farmer's market for local produce, shop online for produce delivery boxes, or grow some of your own. Always choose the freshest-looking produce—avoid anything discolored or wilted, which will have lost vitamins B and C and enzymes.

PANTRY STAPLES FOR < GREEN JUICING >

Although most of your juicing and blending ingredients will be fresh, a few staple additions to your pantry will make your juices even healthier.
Try these:

* Spices, such as ginger, cayenne pepper, turmeric, and cinnamon

* Supplements, such as maca and wheatgrass powder (a high-protein powder)

* Spirulina and chlorella are both chlorophyll-rich and available in powder and pill form

* Nuts, seeds, and nut and seed butters

* Superfoods, such as Manuka honey, coconut, dried acai, and goji berries, raw cacao powder, vanilla beans, hemp seed oil, and seeds

* Long-life versions of rice milk, almond milk, and coconut milk

HINTS AND TIPS

FOR JUICING SUCCESS

NO. 1 KEEPING YOUR PANTRY SUPPLEMENTS FRESH

* Pay attention to any expiration dates and discard out-of-date items
* Store all items in a dry, dark, and preferably cool place, in a sealed container
* Always keep liquid supplements in the refrigerator

NO. 2 GET A GOOD BLEND

* Make sure all your vegetables and fruit are chopped as necessary into similar sizes; soft fruit, such as bananas, can be in larger chunks, while hard items, such as carrots, should be chopped small
* Always use the provided plunger for feeding items into a juicer
* Put solids into a blender bowl and add liquid—don't try to blend without added liquid
* For hard fruit or vegetables, try the highest setting for a smoother blend

NO. 3 PREPPING YOUR VEGETABLES FOR JUICING AND BLENDING

* Wash in cold water to clean—don't soak (you'll lose nutrients)
* For tough-skinned vegetables and fruit and citrus, especially waxed items (unwaxed organic versions are available), peel, core, and/or seed as necessary before juicing
* Some fruit, such as avocados and mangoes, should be pitted because the hard pit will be impossible to pulp

NO. 4 DRINKING YOUR JUICE OR SMOOTHIE

* To retain the most nutrients, drink your prepared juice or smoothie immediately
* Cold-pressed juices tend to store well for longer (24 hours or more), if kept in the refrigerator
* Always use an insulated drink or soup container if you want to blend your juices or smoothies to go—or put a regular travel mug in an insulated bag

NO. 5 MAXIMUM NUTRITION

* To retain as many nutrients as possible, remember juices and blends should never be heated—heating destroys enzymes, vitamin C, and the B-group vitamins
* Cold-press (masticating) juicers may be preferable to centrifugal juicers, which create a lot of heat

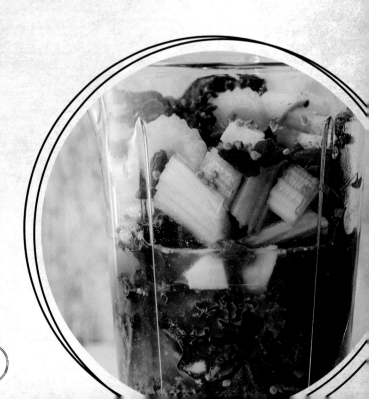

CHOOSING THE RIGHT EQUIPMENT

> YOU'LL GET MAXIMUM ENJOYMENT FROM YOUR JUICING OR BLENDING IF YOU HAVE THE RIGHT EQUIPMENT FOR YOUR NEEDS. OUR EASY GUIDE WILL HELP YOU MAKE THE PERFECT CHOICE.

The first thing to consider is what type of drinks you want to make. Juicers literally extract the juice from produce, either by centrifugal force or various forms of mastication and/or pressing, while blenders simply mash up the produce with added liquid, so you get the whole fruit or veggie in your glass.

> USE OUR AT-A-GLANCE GUIDE TO HELP YOU DECIDE WHICH MACHINE IS RIGHT FOR YOU:

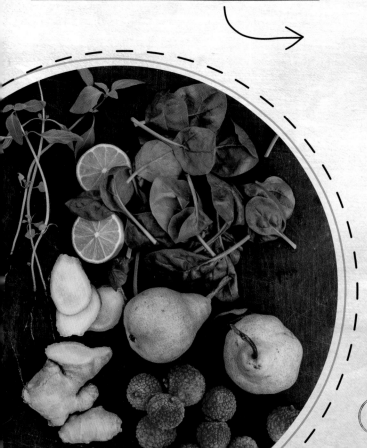

JUICERS

CENTRIFUGAL JUICERS

How they work: Use toothed blades on the bottom of a spinning strainer basket, which separates juice from the pulp by centrifugal force
Best for: All fruit, root vegetables. Less efficient for leaves and herbs
Ease of use: Easy. Some have attachments, such as a citrus juicer, which may be useful
Speed: Usually have at least two speeds
Cleaning: Can be fussy, with up to nine parts
Good to know: The system creates heat, which warms the juice and can reduce the nutritional quality compared with other juicing methods

MASTICATING / COLD-PRESS JUICERS

How they work: Crush the produce using a screw-type system followed by pressing
Best for: All produce—the best machines for extracting juice from leaves and herbs
Ease of use: Reasonable
Speed: Can be time-consuming to set up and slower to juice than centrifugal types
Cleaning: Ideally cleaned straight after use
Good to know: Most research shows they retain more vitamins, plant compounds, and enzymes than centrifugal machines because little heat is produced

MANUAL JUICERS

* You can buy inexpensive manual citrus juicers—a simple cone with a base to collect the juice. You can also purchase manual wheatgrass/leafy greens juicers, ideal if you have a centrifugal juicer.

BLENDERS

FULL-SIZE BLENDERS

How they work: A large jar with steel blades in the bottom attaches to an encased electric motor. Produce is placed in the jar with a liquid; the lid is put on and the blades blend the contents into a thick liquid

Best for: Producing a drink or soup that is fiber-rich and with no waste. Good for crushed-ice smoothies

Ease of use: Easy

Speed: Most blenders come with at least two speeds and a pulse/ice crush option

Cleaning: Easy, although you need to be careful with the blades

Good to know: Smoothie makers are similar to jar blenders but usually include a pouring spout

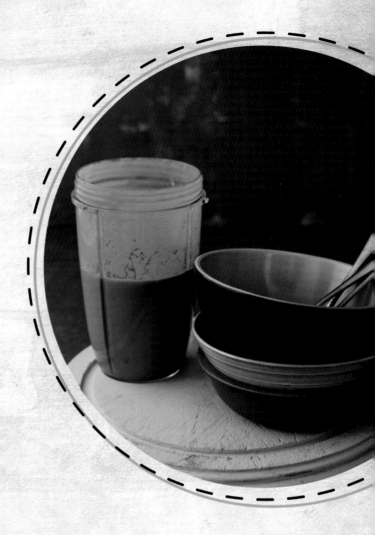

HIGH-SPEED PERSONAL "SUPER" BLENDERS

How they work: Usually use cyclonic action to pulverize and emulsify produce, including tough stems, skins, and seeds, ensuring the nutrients are easily accessed by the digestive system. Like jar blenders, these are ideal for a range of fruit and vegetables, plus liquid. The blended drink is immediately portable, because you can remove the bladed lid and replace it with a standard spill-proof lid

Best for: All types of fruit and vegetables and for maximizing nutrients

Ease of use: Designed to be especially user-friendly, with a quickly removed bladed lid and clever upside-down blending/drinking cup design

Speed: The more expensive versions are especially fast

Cleaning: Easy

Good to know: These new-wave blenders are ideal for singles and people on the go, because there is no need to transfer the blended recipe into a different container. They also usually come with a milling blade for chopping nuts, grains, and seeds

IMMERSION HAND BLENDERS

How they work: A blending blade is housed in an electric handheld wand and is used directly in your own pitcher, mug, or bowl, or a jar may be supplied

Best for: Softer fruit and vegetables and items chopped small. Great for single servings, shots, and quick soup blends

Ease of use: Easy to hold and use but taller, narrower bowls are preferable to wide and shallow ones, which can mean the contents spill out during blending

Speed: Usually one speed

Cleaning: Easy

Good to know: Though not as versatile as other blenders, these can be inexpensive and are ideal standbys for small kitchens, basic soft-fruit blends, and people in a hurry

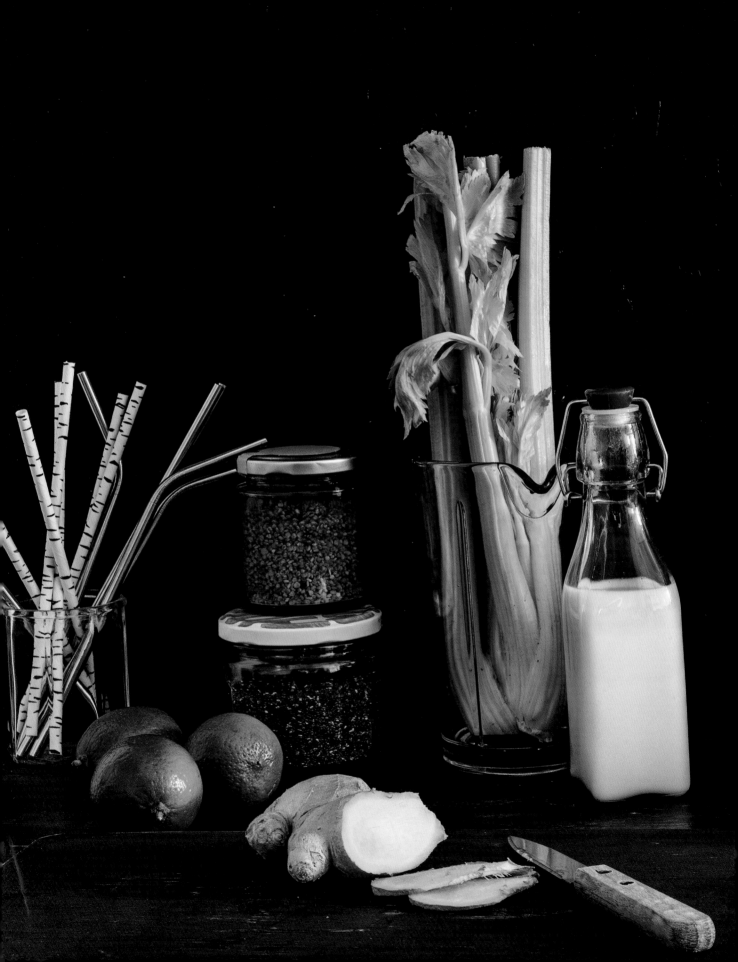

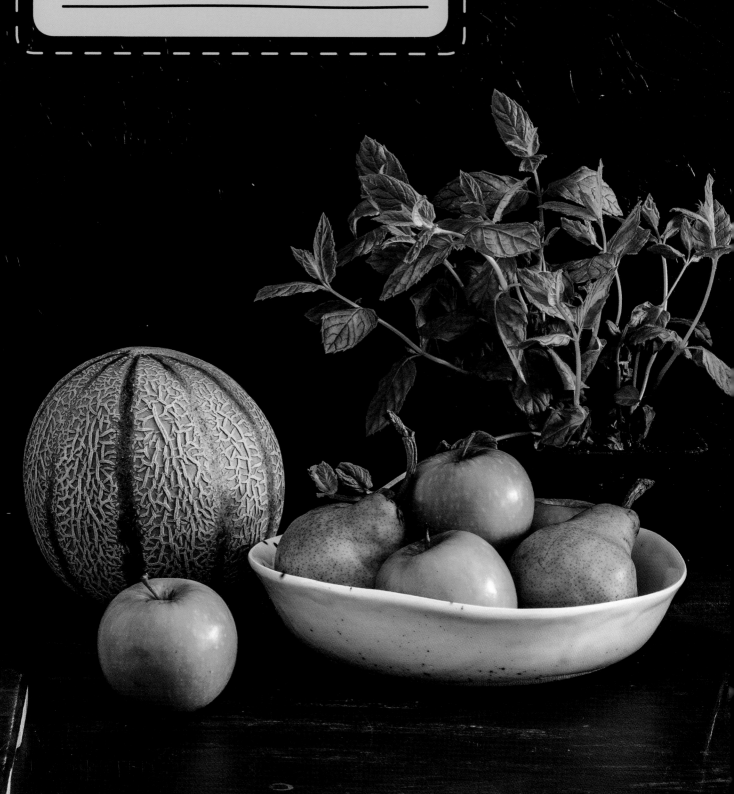

GREEN TO
CLEANSE

GREEN ENVY

SERVES 1

YOUR FRIENDS WILL BE GREEN WITH ENVY WHEN THEY SEE THE YOUTHFUL NEW YOU GLOWING WITH HEALTH AND FULL OF ENERGY.

Ingredients

1 GREEN APPLE

4 CELERY STALKS, PLUS EXTRA TO GARNISH

½ CUCUMBER

3 ½ cups SPINACH

⅓ cup FRESH MINT

1 teaspoon chlorophyll powder

ice cubes, to serve (optional)

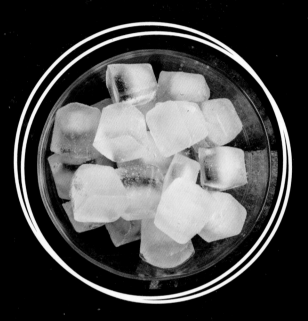

MAKE THIS JUICE

- COARSELY CHOP THE APPLE, CELERY, AND CUCUMBER.

- PUT THE SPINACH, MINT, APPLE, CELERY, AND CUCUMBER INTO THE JUICER FUNNEL AND JUICE.

- STIR IN THE CHLOROPHYLL POWDER UNTIL COMBINED. FILL A GLASS WITH ICE, POUR IN THE JUICE, AND SERVE IMMEDIATELY, GARNISHED WITH A TRIMMED CELERY STALK.

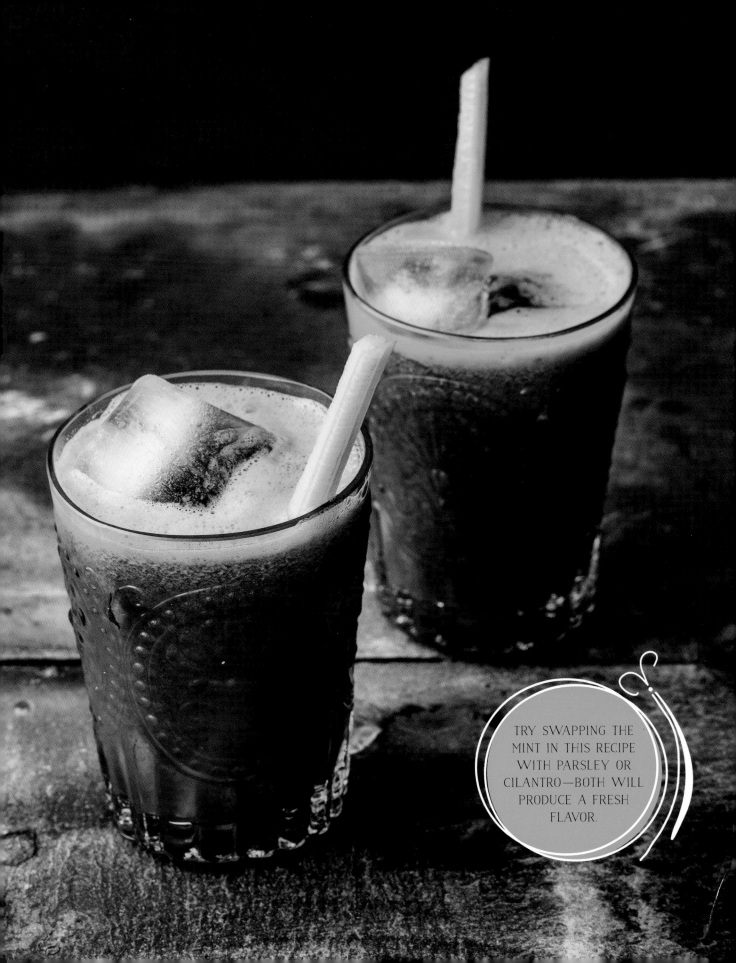

TRY SWAPPING THE
MINT IN THIS RECIPE
WITH PARSLEY OR
CILANTRO—BOTH WILL
PRODUCE A FRESH
FLAVOR.

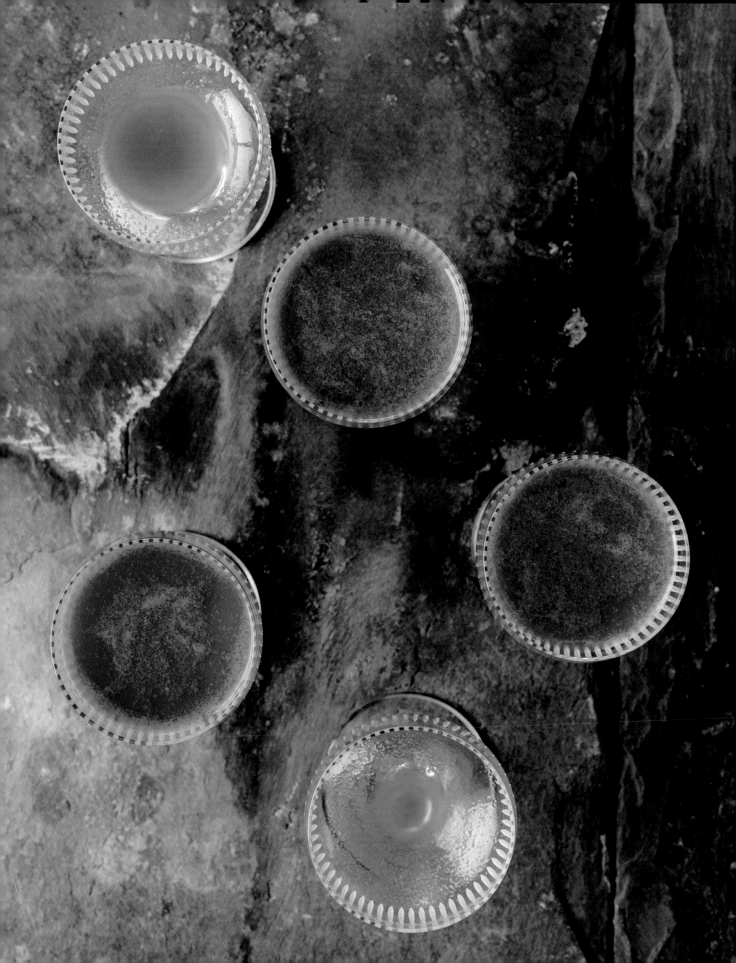

GREEN CLEANER

THINK OF THIS SMOOTHIE AS A HUG FROM THE INSIDE OUT. IT LOOKS AND TASTES GOOD, AND IS PACKED WITH VITAMINS A, B, C, AND E, PLUS IRON AND POTASSIUM.

SERVES 1

Ingredients

1 APPLE, HALVED

½ CUP COARSELY CHOPPED GREEN CURLY KALE

2 KIWIS, PEELED

2 FLAT-LEAF PARSLEY SPRIGS

½ AVOCADO, PITTED AND FLESH SCOOPED FROM SKIN

¼ cup chilled water

small handful crushed ice

ENHANCE THE PURIFYING QUALITY OF THIS SMOOTHIE WITH A SQUEEZE OF LIME.

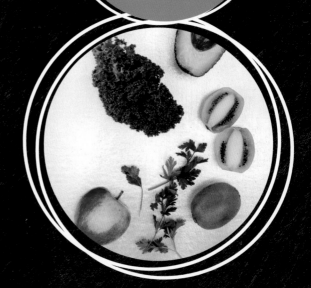

MIX IT UP

- FEED THE APPLE, KALE, AND KIWIS THROUGH A JUICER.

- POUR THE JUICE INTO A BLENDER, ADD THE PARSLEY AND AVOCADO, THEN BLEND.

- ADD THE WATER AND CRUSHED ICE AND BLEND AGAIN UNTIL SMOOTH.

- POUR INTO A GLASS AND SERVE IMMEDIATELY.

MELON & COCONUT MOJITO

THIS FRESH AND FRUITY SMOOTHIE WILL BRING BACK HAPPY MEMORIES OF SUMMER DAYS.

SERVES 1

Ingredients

¾ CUP SPINACH

⅔ CUP COCONUT FLESH

1 cup chilled water

⅔ CUP PEELED AND SEEDED CANTALOUPE CHUNKS

1 tablespoon CHOPPED FRESH MINT

juice of ½ lime

⅓ CUP PEELED AND PITTED MANGO SLICES

crushed ice, to serve (optional)

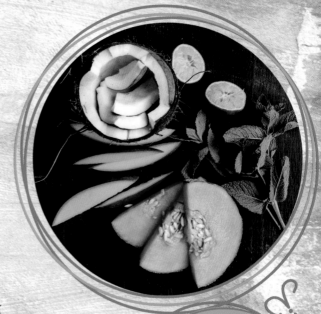

YOU CAN SWAP THE CANTALOUPE WITH HONEYDEW MELON, IF PREFERRED.

GET BLENDING

- PUT THE SPINACH, COCONUT, AND WATER INTO A BLENDER, AND BLEND UNTIL SMOOTH.

- ADD THE MELON, MINT, LIME JUICE, AND MANGO, AND BLEND UNTIL SMOOTH AND CREAMY. POUR OVER CRUSHED ICE, IF USING, AND SERVE IMMEDIATELY.

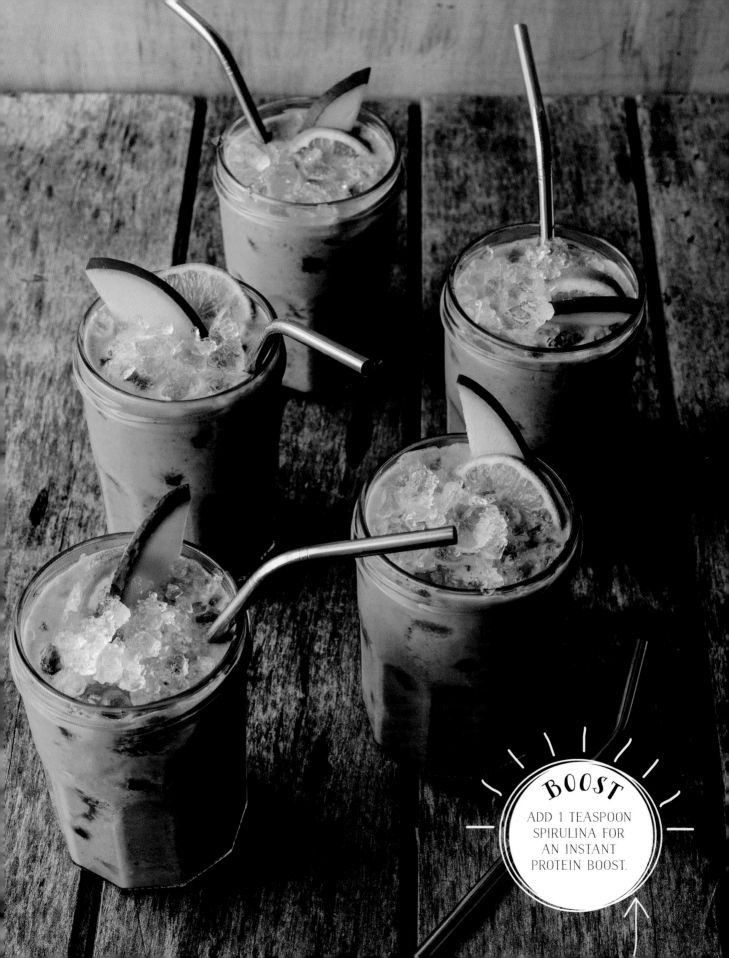

BOOST

ADD 1 TEASPOON SPIRULINA FOR AN INSTANT PROTEIN BOOST.

DR. GREEN

Ingredients

1 cup ARUGULA

1 tablespoon CHOPPED FRESH MINT

1 cup chilled water

¾ CUP PEELED AND SEEDED
HONEYDEW MELON CHUNKS

1½ teaspoons chlorophyll powder

juice of ½ lemon

1-inch PIECE FRESH GINGER, PEELED

4 ice cubes

>BLEND IT<

- PUT THE ARUGULA, MINT, AND WATER INTO A BLENDER, AND BLEND UNTIL SMOOTH.

- ADD THE MELON, CHLOROPHYLL POWDER, LEMON JUICE, GINGER, AND ICE CUBES, AND BLEND AGAIN UNTIL SMOOTH AND CREAMY.

LAVENDER BOOST

SERVES 1

Ingredients

½ LARGE FENNEL BULB

½ HEAD ROMAINE LETTUCE

1 cup PEELED, SEEDED HONEYDEW
MELON CHUNKS

1 lime, quartered

5 LAVENDER FLOWER STEMS

MIX IT<

- COARSELY CHOP THE FENNEL AND LETTUCE SO THEY WILL FIT INTO THE JUICER.

- FEED THE FENNEL, LETTUCE, MELON, AND LIME INTO THE FUNNEL OF THE JUICER WITH THE LAVENDER AND JUICE. STIR WELL AND SERVE IMMEDIATELY.

DR. GREEN

LAVENDER CAN BE AN OVERPOWERING FLAVOR, SO USE IT SPARINGLY. YOU CAN USE DRIED LAVENDER, BUT REMEMBER THAT THE POTENCY INCREASES WITH DRYING.

BOOST

ADD 2 TEASPOONS BEE POLLEN TO HELP FIGHT OFF FATIGUE.

LAVENDER BOOST

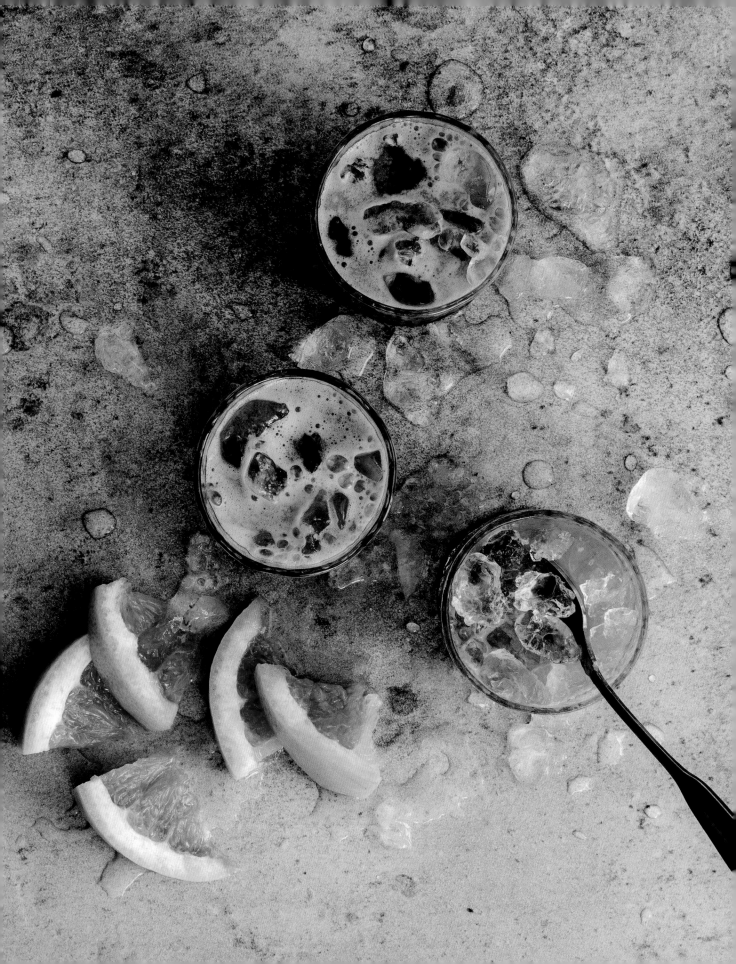

GRAPEFRUIT CRUSH

SERVES 1   THIS FRESH AND COOLING JUICE IS MIXED WITH COCONUT WATER, WHICH IS PACKED WITH ELECTROLYTES AND MINERALS TO HELP COUNTER DEHYDRATION.

Ingredients

½ CUCUMBER

½ PINK GRAPEFRUIT, PLUS EXTRA SEGMENTS TO GARNISH

2 KIWIS

2 CELERY STALKS

1 teaspoon maca powder

¼ cup coconut water

crushed ice, to serve (optional)

CHANGE IT UP
Substitute a flavored coconut water, such as coconut water with passion fruit or acai.

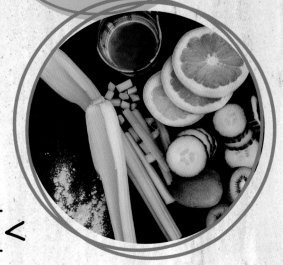

>GO CRUSH CRAZY!<

- COARSELY CHOP THE CUCUMBER, GRAPEFRUIT, KIWIS, AND CELERY. PUT INTO THE FUNNEL OF THE JUICER AND JUICE.

- STIR IN THE MACA POWDER AND COCONUT WATER UNTIL COMBINED, THEN POUR OVER CRUSHED ICE, IF USING. GARNISH WITH GRAPEFRUIT SEGMENTS AND SERVE IMMEDIATELY.

MELON, PEAR & GINGER SPRITZER

A REFRESHINGLY HEALTHY VERSION OF GINGER BEER WITH NO CHEMICALS AND NO ADDED SUGARS, JUST 100 PERCENT NATURAL INGREDIENTS.

SERVES 1

Ingredients

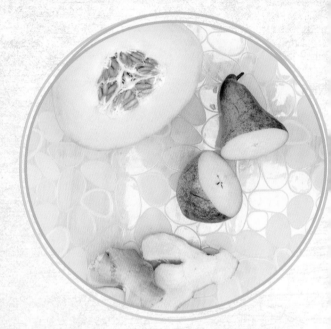

½ HONEYDEW MELON, PEELED AND THICKLY SLICED

½-inch PIECE FRESH GINGER

1 PEAR, HALVED

Small handful ice (optional)

½ CUP sparkling mineral water, chilled

TIME FOR A SPRITZ

- FEED THE MELON, GINGER, AND PEAR THROUGH A JUICER.

- FILL A GLASS HALFWAY WITH ICE, IF USING, THEN POUR IN THE JUICE.

- FILL WITH THE SPARKLING MINERAL WATER AND SERVE IMMEDIATELY.

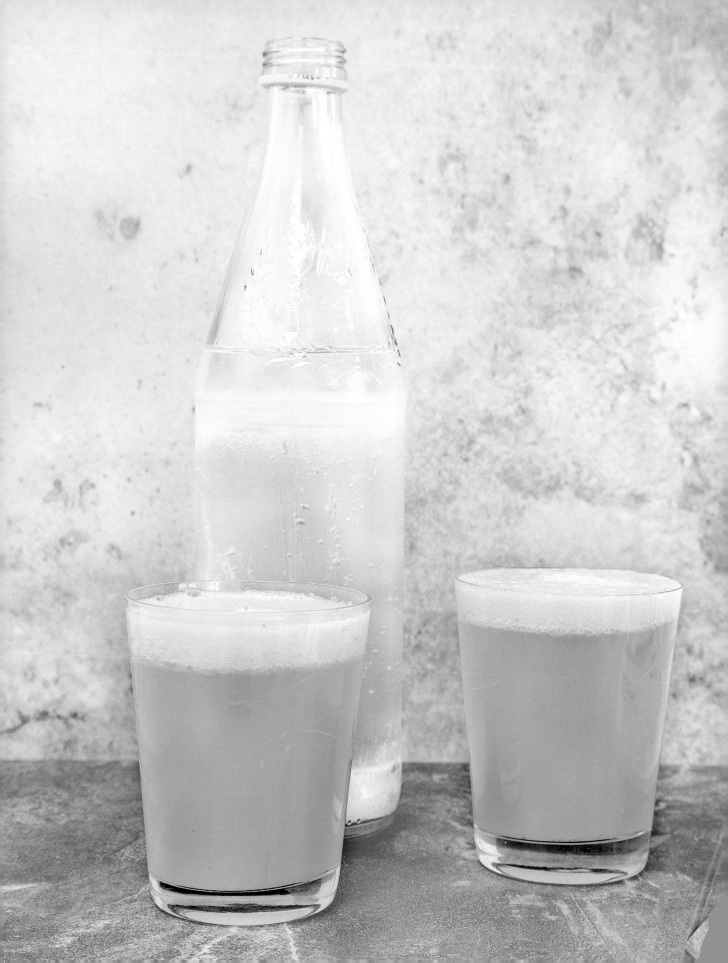

REVITALIZE
YOUR BODY WITH
ALKALIZING GREENS

ONE OF THE MANY REASONS GREEN JUICES ARE SUPER-HEALTHY IS THAT THEY ARE ALKALINE. THIS MEANS THEY HELP COMBAT THE EFFECTS OF AN OVERACIDIC DIET, HELP TO DETOXIFY OUR SYSTEMS, AND KEEP US IN GOOD GENERAL HEALTH.

DID YOU KNOW that most of us eat a diet that is really high in acidic foods? Meat, cheese, refined cereals, alcohol, and low-quality foods high in sugar and processed fats all create an internal acidic environment. Although the kidneys are capabale of removing excess acid naturally, our modern diet could easily overload them. Many leading nutritionists believe this can result in a whole host of health problems, partly because the kidneys try to redress the acid balance by "robbing" us of important minerals, such as magnesium, calcium, and potassium, which are vital for acid excretion. With these minerals depleted, we find it harder to make hormones, enzymes, and neurotransmitters necessary for energy and for fighting infection and inflammation.

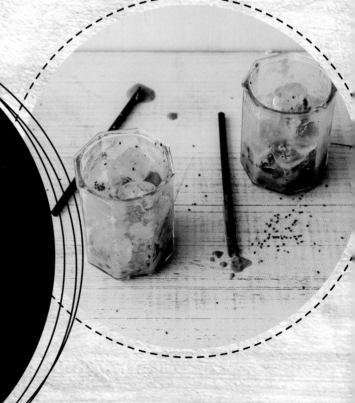

HERE ARE SOME SIGNS YOUR BODY MAY BE OVERACIDIC:

- Frequent colds or flu
- Low energy, chronic fatigue, poor sleep quality
- Aching muscles; back pain
- Joint pain, osteoarthritis, osteoporosis
- Bladder and kidney problems
- Acne, eczema, or psoriasis
- Lack of concentration, headaches
- Bloating and weight gain
- Mood swings. PMS

The good news is that you can easily create a more alkaline environment for your body by eating fewer acidic foods.

ADJUSTING YOUR PH BALANCE

Your body's acid/alkaline balance is also known as its pH balance. pH is measured on a scale of 0–14, with 0 being highly acidic and 14 highly alkaline. Apart from our stomach acid, which needs to be high to break down the food we eat, the optimum pH in the rest of the body should be about 7.4. In general, a diet high in vegetables and fruit helps alkalize us, while a diet high in protein, particularly animal protein, refined cereals, sugars, and processed foods, increases our acidity. Clinical trials have proved that an alkaline body is healthier than an acidic body, and experts believe a good balance is 70–80 percent alkaline-forming foods to 20–30 percent acid-forming, but most of us have exactly the reverse balance.

Most people find that when they switch to a high alkaline diet, symptoms such as those listed opposite improve quickly. Juicing and blending are ideal ways to maximize the alkalizing effects of foods, because of the concentrated nutrition they provide and because the juicing/blending process breaks down food and helps nutrient absorption in our bodies. Juices and blends are also high in water, which has an almost perfect neutral pH of 7.

HIGH ALKALINE-FORMING FOODS:

Leafy greens, other greens, avocados, tomatoes, many fruits—especially lemons, limes, melons, grapefruit, grapes, papaya, and kiwi—herbs, most spices, apple cider vinegar, soy, almonds. Supplements, such as wheatgrass, chia seeds, and chlorella, are highly alkaline.

HIGH ACID-FORMING FOODS:

Animal proteins—including beef, lamb, pork, chicken, shellfish, duck, eggs, and dairy produce—refined cereals, caffeine, sugar, carbonated drinks, alcohol, and processed foods.

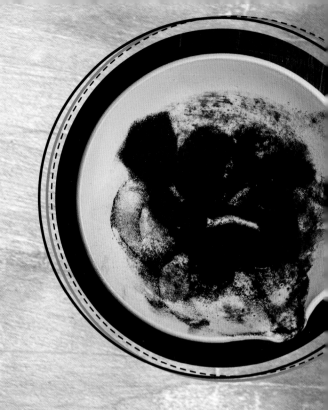

CHLOROPHYLL

WHAT IT IS AND HOW THE PIGMENT POSITIVELY AFFECTS OUR HEALTH

Chlorophyll is the dark-green pigment found in plants and algae. Abundant in leafy greens and herbs, wheatgrass, and in the algae supplement chlorella, chlorophyll is not only highly alkaline, it is also rich in vitamins, minerals, plant compounds, and antioxidants. It may help to increase the quality and quantity of our red blood cells and, as a result, may increase our oxygen levels, improve energy, enhance well-being, and stimulate the immune system.

Chlorophyll is a clinically proven anti-inflammatory and can help protect us against diseases, such as rheumatoid arthritis, heart disease, and certain digestive disorders, including inflammatory bowel disease (IBS). In other words, increasing the amount of chlorophyll in your diet may be one of the best things you can do to keep your pH in balance and yourself feeling great.

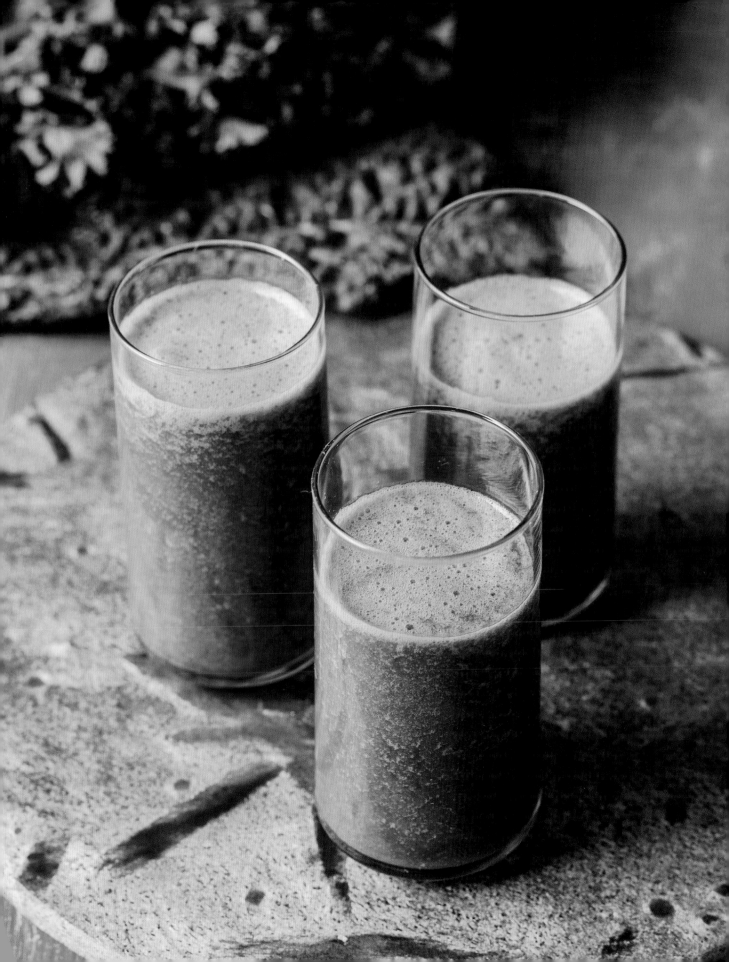

ALOE REFRESHER

ALOE VERA IS PACKED WITH VITAMINS AND MINERALS. IT CAN AID DIGESTION AND DETOXIFICATION AND BOOST THE IMMUNE SYSTEM, SO IT IS A GREAT ADDITION TO YOUR GREEN JUICES AND SMOOTHIES.

SERVES 1

Ingredients

½ cup SHREDDED KALE

1 cup chilled water

⅔ cup SEEDED AND PEELED WATERMELON CHUNKS

½ cup PEELED AND PITTED MANGO CHUNKS

1-2 tablespoons aloe vera gel, to taste

1 teaspoon wheatgrass powder

4 ice cubes

TIP
Aloe vera has a strong flavor, so use less until you're used to the taste.

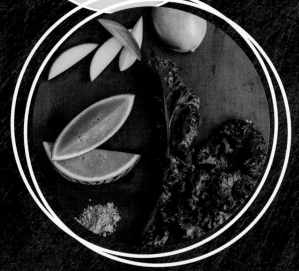

BLEND IT

- ADD THE KALE TO THE BLENDER WITH THE WATER AND BLEND UNTIL SMOOTH.

- ADD THE WATERMELON AND MANGO CHUNKS TO THE BLENDER.

- ADD THE ALOE VERA GEL, WHEATGRASS POWDER, AND ICE CUBES, AND BLEND UNTIL SMOOTH.

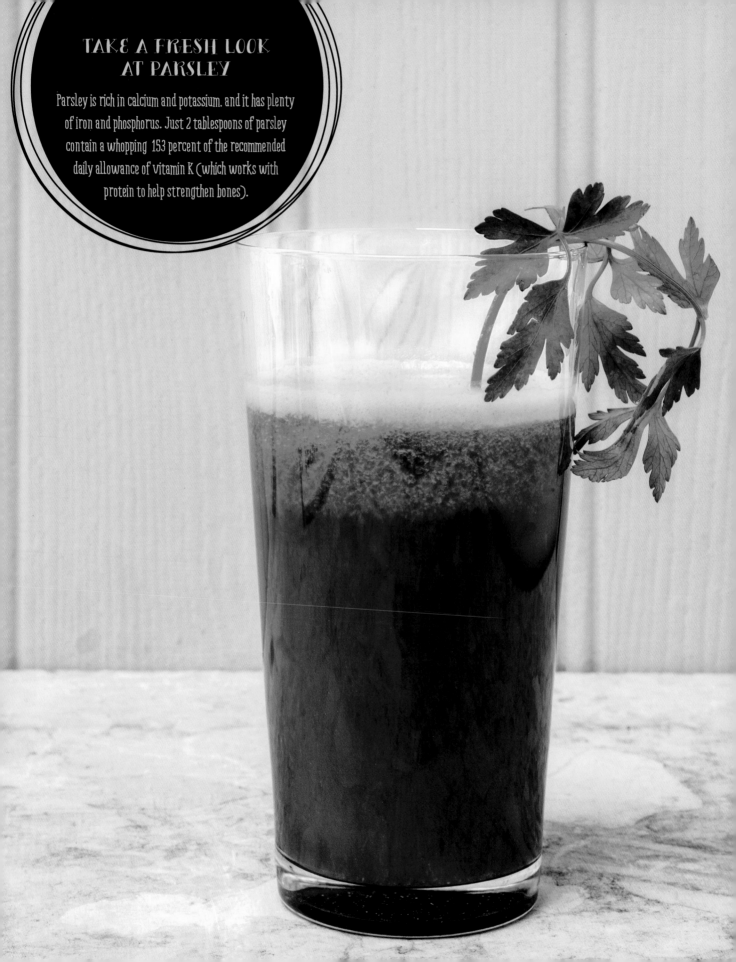

PARSLEY PURIFIER

SERVES 1 AS A DIURETIC, THIS DRINK REALLY HELPS TO CLEANSE YOUR BODY. THE STRONG FLAVORS OF THE HERBS AND GARLIC ARE BALANCED BY THE NATURAL SWEETNESS OF THE SUGAR SNAP PEAS AND THE DELICATE FLAVOR OF THE CUCUMBER.

Ingredients

1½ CUPS SUGAR SNAP PEAS

SMALL HANDFUL FRESH FLAT-LEAF PARSLEY

2 STEMS FRESH ROSEMARY

1 GARLIC CLOVE

2 CUPS YOUNG SPINACH

½ CUCUMBER

2 CELERY STICKS, HALVED

1 teaspoon hemp oil

chilled water, to taste

ice, to serve (optional)

GIVE IT A WHIRL

- FEED THE SUGAR SNAP PEAS, PARSLEY (RESERVING 1 STEM TO GARNISH), ROSEMARY, AND GARLIC INTO A JUICER, FOLLOWED BY THE SPINACH, CUCUMBER, AND CELERY.

- POUR INTO A GLASS, STIR IN THE HEMP OIL AND WATER TO TASTE, THEN GARNISH WITH THE PARSLEY STEM AND SERVE WITH ICE, IF USING.

GREEN CRUSH

HAVEN'T TRIED KOHLRABI BEFORE? THIS IS YOUR CHANCE—ITS CRUNCHY TEXTURE AND MILD SPICE WORK WELL WITH GENTLE FLAVORS SO IT ISN'T OVERPOWERING.

SERVES 1

Ingredients

1 CUP PEELED, CHOPPED KOHLRABI

¾ CUP CHOPPED ZUCCHINI

⅔ cup chilled water

½ cup coconut milk

½ AVOCADO, PITTED AND FLESH FLESH SCOOPED FROM SKIN

juice of ½ lime

4 ice cubes

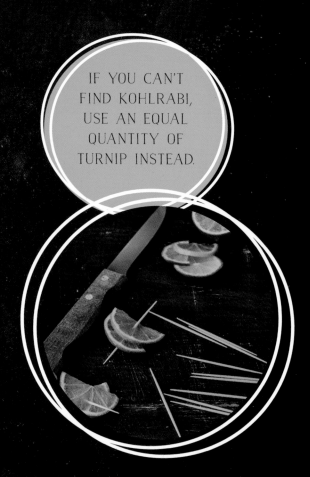

IF YOU CAN'T FIND KOHLRABI, USE AN EQUAL QUANTITY OF TURNIP INSTEAD.

BLEND IT!

- ADD THE CHOPPED KOHLRABI AND ZUCCHINI TO A BLENDER WITH THE WATER AND COCONUT MILK, AND BLEND UNTIL SMOOTH AND CREAMY.

- CHOP THE AVOCADO, ADD TO THE BLENDER WITH THE LIME JUICE AND ICE CUBES, AND BLEND AGAIN UNTIL SMOOTH. SERVE IMMEDIATELY.

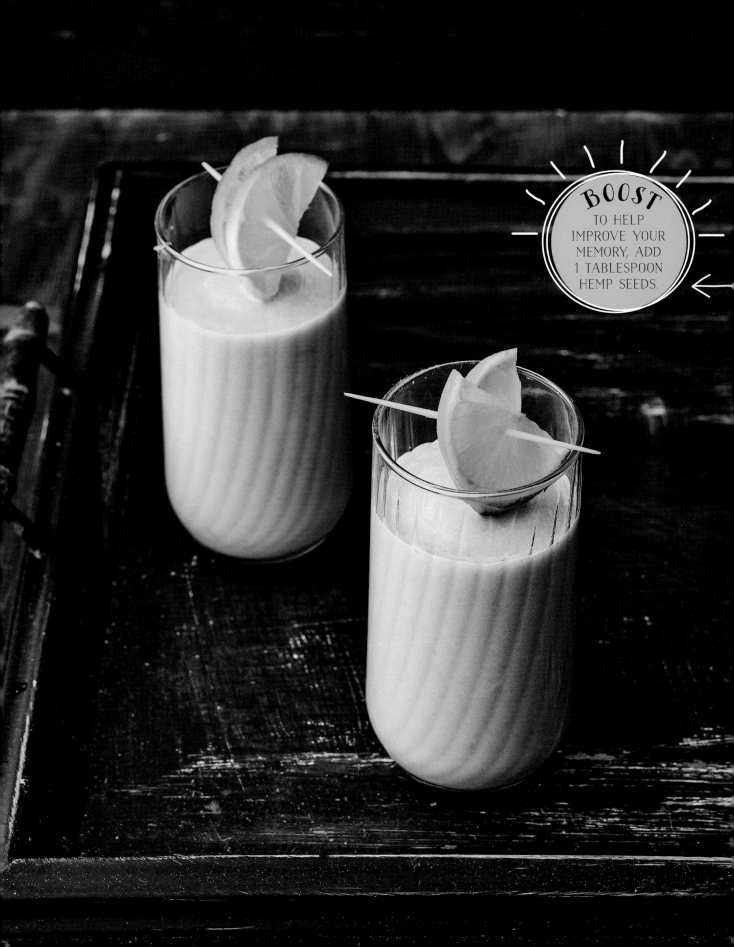

BOOST
TO HELP
IMPROVE YOUR
MEMORY, ADD
1 TABLESPOON
HEMP SEEDS.

COOL AS A CUCUMBER

SERVES 1

THIS IS LIKE A COOLING SUMMER SALAD IN A GLASS—LIGHT AND FRESH, WITH A GENTLE PEPPERINESS FROM THE ARUGULA, A DASH OF MOUTH-FRESHENING GARDEN MINT, AND A HINT OF APPLEY SWEETNESS.

Ingredients

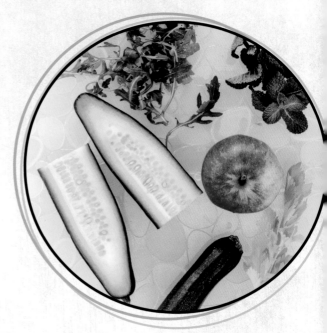

½ CUCUMBER, HALVED

½ CUP ARUGULA

3 STEMS FRESH MINT

1 ZUCCHINI

1 CELERY STALK, HALVED

1 APPLE, HALVED

small handful crushed ice (optional)

>GO CUCUMBER CRAZY!<

- FEED THE CUCUMBER, ARUGULA, AND MINT INTO A JUICER, FOLLOWED BY THE ZUCCHINI, CELERY, AND APPLE.

- FILL A GLASS HALFWAY WITH CRUSHED ICE, IF USING, THEN POUR IN THE JUICE AND SERVE IMMEDIATELY.

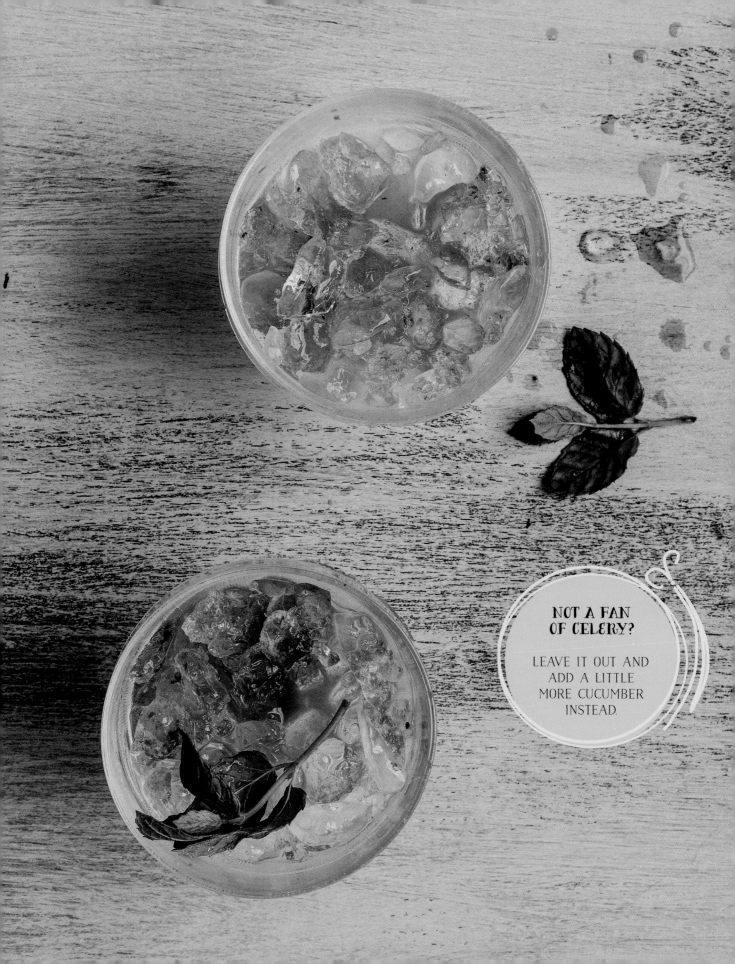

NOT A FAN
OF CELERY?

LEAVE IT OUT AND
ADD A LITTLE
MORE CUCUMBER
INSTEAD.

FLU SHOT

SERVES 1

> FRESH AND PUNCHY, THIS VIBRANT SHOT WILL GIVE YOU AN INSTANT CLEANSE.

Ingredients

½ GREEN APPLE, PEELED AND CORED

1½ tablespoons FRESH PARSLEY, PLUS A SMALL SPRIG TO GARNISH

⅙ CUCUMBER

PINCH OF CAYENNE PEPPER

3 ½ tablespoons chilled water

> GO EASY ON THE CAYENNE PEPPER—YOU CAN ALWAYS ADD MORE BUT YOU CAN'T TAKE IT OUT.

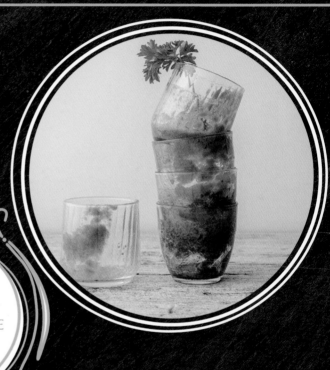

MAKE IT SMOOTH

- PUT THE APPLE, PARSLEY, CUCUMBER, AND CAYENNE PEPPER INTO A BLENDER.

- POUR IN THE WATER AND BLEND UNTIL SMOOTH. SERVE IMMEDIATELY.

GREEN TROPICS

SERVES 1

FULL OF BURSTING TROPICAL FLAVOR, THIS SHOT WILL GIVE YOU AN IMMEDIATE LIFT.

AS YOU GET USED TO THE FLAVOR OF WHEATGRASS, INCREASE THE AMOUNT TO 1 TEASPOON.

Ingredients

2 tablespoons SHREDDED KALE

½ CUP PEELED PINEAPPLE CHUNKS, PLUS A SMALL SEGMENT TO GARNISH

½ CUP SPINACH

½ teaspoon wheatgrass powder

3 ½ tablespoons chilled water

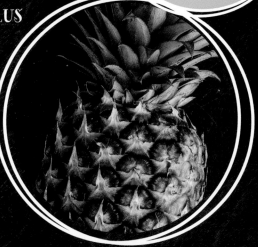

READY SET ... BLEND

- ADD THE KALE AND PINEAPPLE TO A BLENDER WITH THE SPINACH AND WHEATGRASS POWDER.

  POUR IN THE WATER AND BLEND UNTIL SMOOTH.
- SERVE IMMEDIATELY.

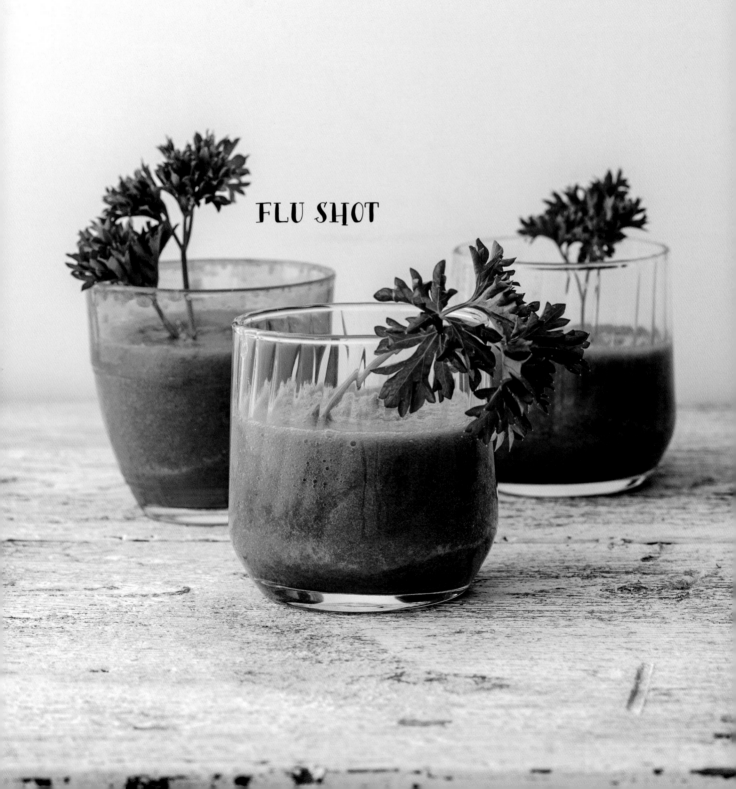

FLU SHOT

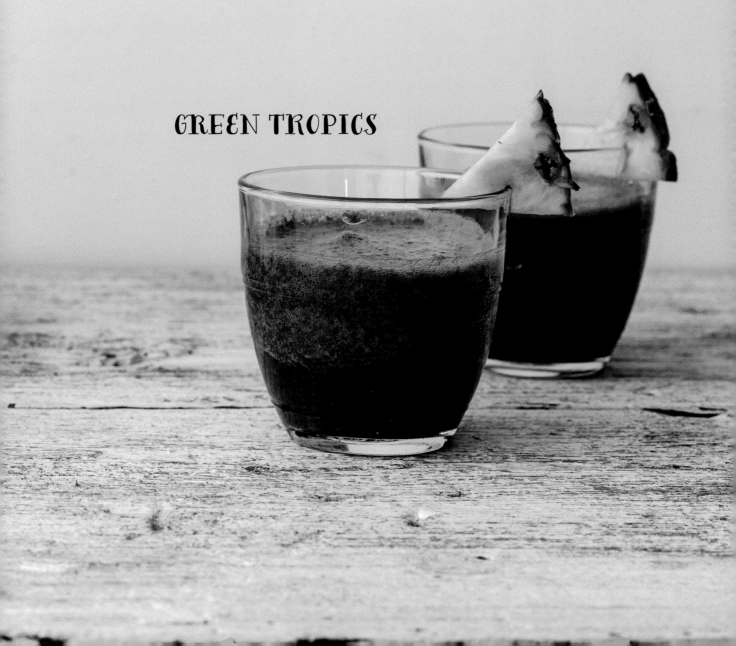

BOOST

ADD 1 TEASPOON CHLOROPHYLL POWDER TO AID LIVER AND COLON CLEANSING.

SEE GREEN TROPICS P. 35

GREEN TROPICS

KEEN GREEN SOUP

THIS SIMPLE, INVIGORATING SOUP WILL COOL YOU DOWN ON A HOT DAY.

Ingredients

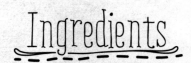

½ CUCUMBER

2 CELERY STALKS

2 tablespoons CHOPPED FRESH PARSLEY, PLUS EXTRA TO GARNISH

2 tablespoons CHOPPED FRESH MINT

2 tablespoons CHOPPED FRESH CILANTRO

1 cup chilled water

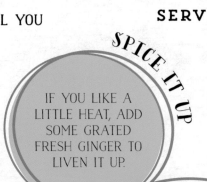

SPICE IT UP

IF YOU LIKE A LITTLE HEAT, ADD SOME GRATED FRESH GINGER TO LIVEN IT UP.

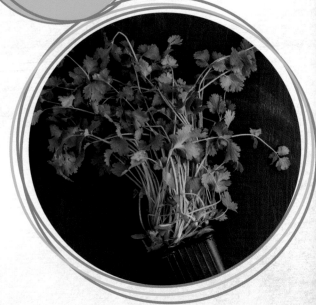

CHILL OUT

- CHOP THE CUCUMBER AND CELERY AND ADD TO A BLENDER WITH THE PARSLEY, MINT, CILANTRO, AND WATER. BLEND UNTIL SMOOTH.

- SERVE IMMEDIATELY OR CHILL IN THE REFRIGERATOR AND STIR JUST BEFORE SERVING. GARNISH WITH PARSLEY.

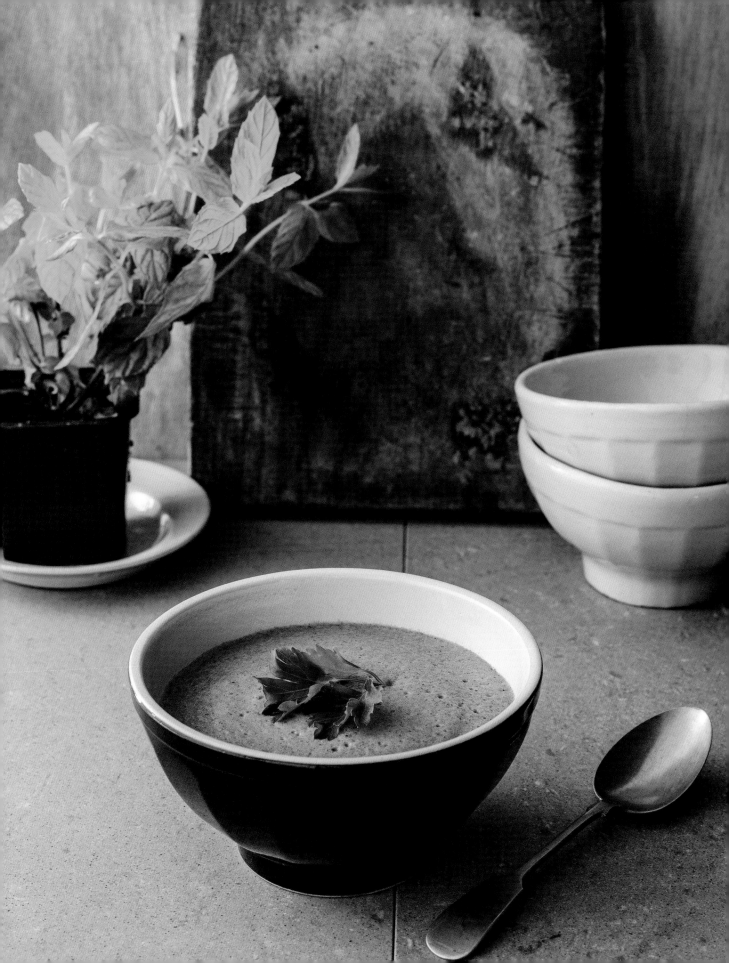

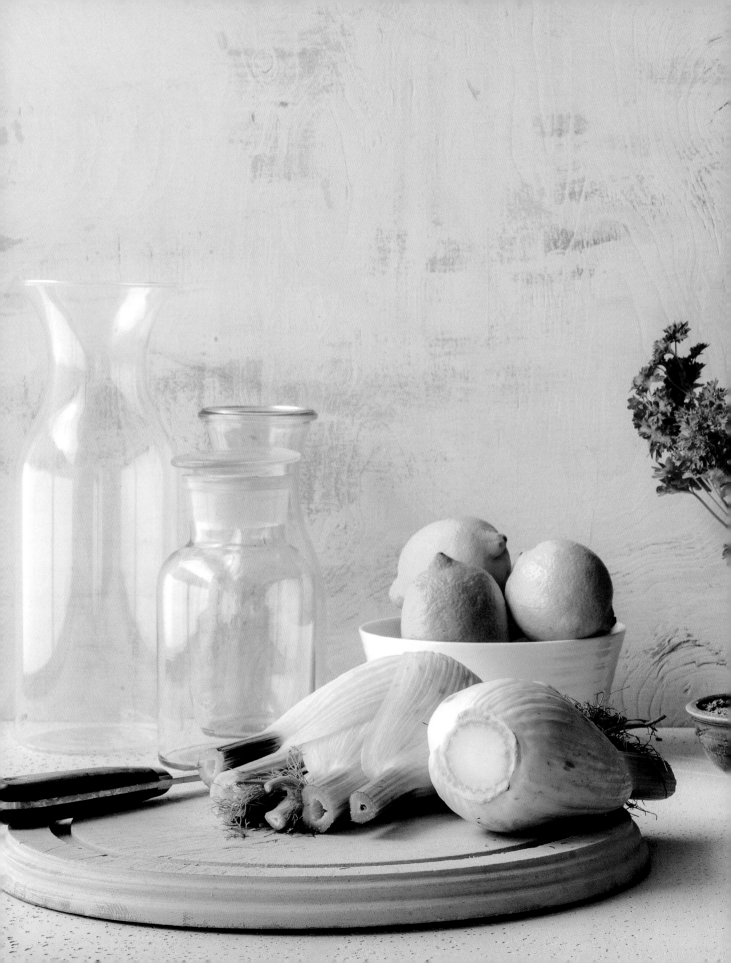

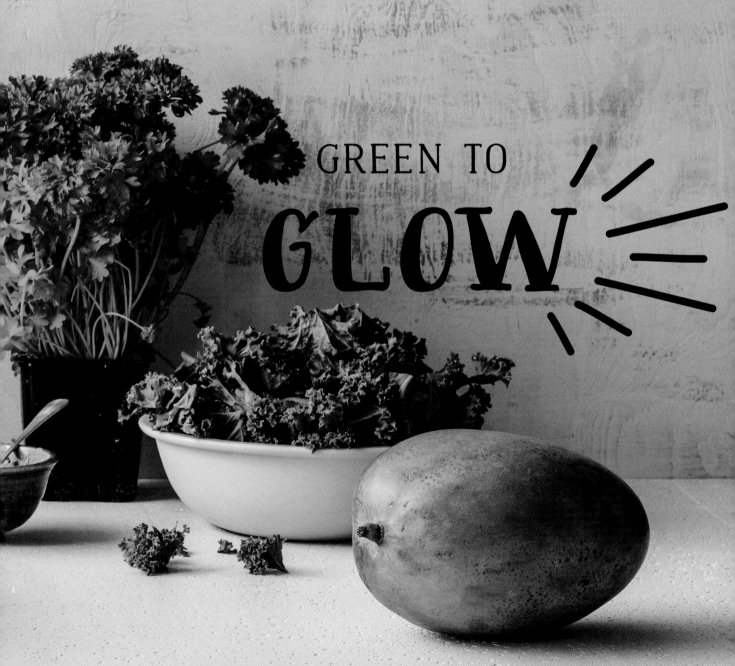

GREEN TO
GLOW

DANDELION COOLER

DANDELIONS HAVE A LONG LIST OF HEALTH BENEFITS, INCLUDING TREATING SKIN CONDITIONS. IF YOU DON'T USE WEED KILLERS, YOU CAN FORAGE FOR THEM IN YOUR OWN YARD FROM SPRING.

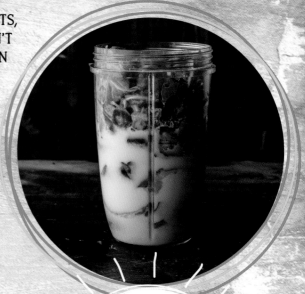

Ingredients

½ CUP DANDELION GREENS

10 SPRIGS WATERCRESS

1 CUP chilled water

1 LARGE PEAR

3½ tablespoons coconut milk

ice cubes, to serve (optional)

BOOST

ADD 1 TEASPOON MACA POWDER TO HELP CLEAR ACNE AND BLEMISHES.

>SMOOTH BLEND<

- PUT THE DANDELION GREENS, WATERCRESS, AND WATER INTO A BLENDER AND BLEND UNTIL SMOOTH.

- CHOP AND SEED THE PEAR AND ADD IT TO THE BLENDER WITH THE COCONUT MILK, THEN BLEND AGAIN UNTIL SMOOTH AND CREAMY.

- STIR WELL, POUR OVER ICE, IF USING, AND SERVE IMMEDIATELY.

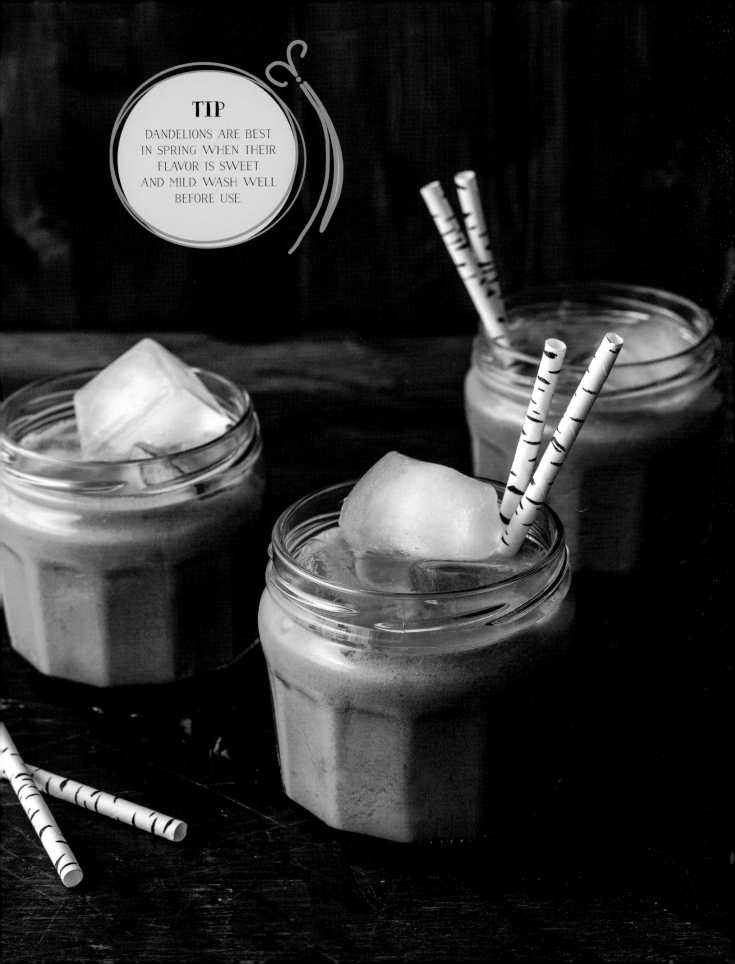

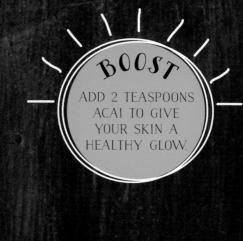

BOOST

ADD 2 TEASPOONS
ACAI TO GIVE
YOUR SKIN A
HEALTHY GLOW.

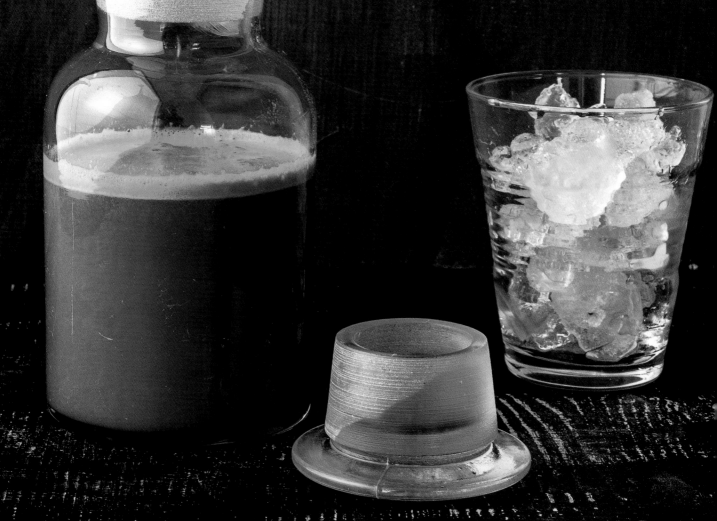

FENNEL FLUSH

SERVES 1

FENNEL IS A GREAT SOURCE OF FIBER AND HAS POTENT ANTIOXIDANTS, WHICH HAVE BEEN SHOWN TO REDUCE INFLAMMATION. TAKING CARE OF YOUR INSIDES WILL SOON HAVE YOU GLOWING ON THE OUTSIDE.

Celery is a good substitute for fennel. but you will lose the slight licorice flavor.

Ingredients

1 LARGE FENNEL BULB

1 GREEN APPLE

1 LIME

3 ½ CUPS SPINACH

½ CUP FRESH MINT

FENNEL LEAVES, TO GARNISH

crushed ice, to serve (optional)

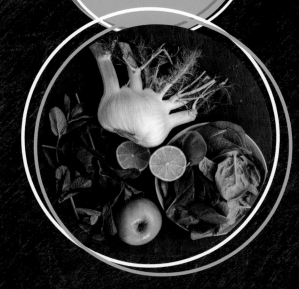

MIX IT UP

- COARSELY CHOP THE FENNEL AND APPLE AND CUT THE LIME INTO QUARTERS.

- FEED THE SPINACH, MINT, FENNEL, APPLE, AND LIME INTO THE FUNNEL OF A JUICER AND JUICE.

- STIR WELL AND POUR OVER THE CRUSHED ICE, IF USING. GARNISH WITH FEATHERY FENNEL LEAVES AND SERVE IMMEDIATELY.

MUSCULAR MAGIC

THIS SMOOTHIE CONTAINS A GOOD DOSE OF LEAFY GREENS, PLENTY OF HEALTHY MONOUNSATURATED FATS FROM THE AVOCADO, AND PROTEIN FROM THE NUTS—IT'S ALMOST A MEAL IN A GLASS.

SERVES 1

Ingredients

¾ CUP CHOPPED GREEN CURLY KALE

SMALL HANDFUL FRESH FLAT-LEAF PARSLEY

½ ROMAINE LETTUCE

2 CELERY STALKS, HALVED

1 APPLE, HALVED

½ LEMON

⅓ CUP SLIVERED ALMONDS

½ AVOCADO, PITTED AND FLESH SCOOPED FROM SKIN

small handful crushed ice

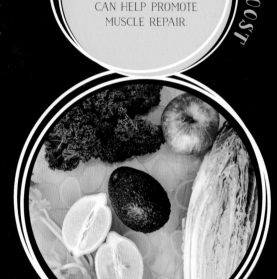

POSTEXERCISE BOOST

HAVING A HEALTHY SNACK SUCH AS THIS SMOOTHIE WITHIN 30 MINUTES OF EXERCISE CAN HELP PROMOTE MUSCLE REPAIR.

WHIZ IT

- FEED THE KALE, PARSLEY, AND LETTUCE THROUGH A JUICER, FOLLOWED BY THE CELERY, APPLE, AND LEMON.

- PUT THE ALMONDS INTO A BLENDER AND BLEND UNTIL FINELY GROUND.

- ADD THE KALE JUICE MIX AND AVOCADO FLESH, THEN BLEND AGAIN UNTIL SMOOTH.

- ADD THE CRUSHED ICE AND BLEND AGAIN. POUR INTO A GLASS AND SERVE IMMEDIATELY.

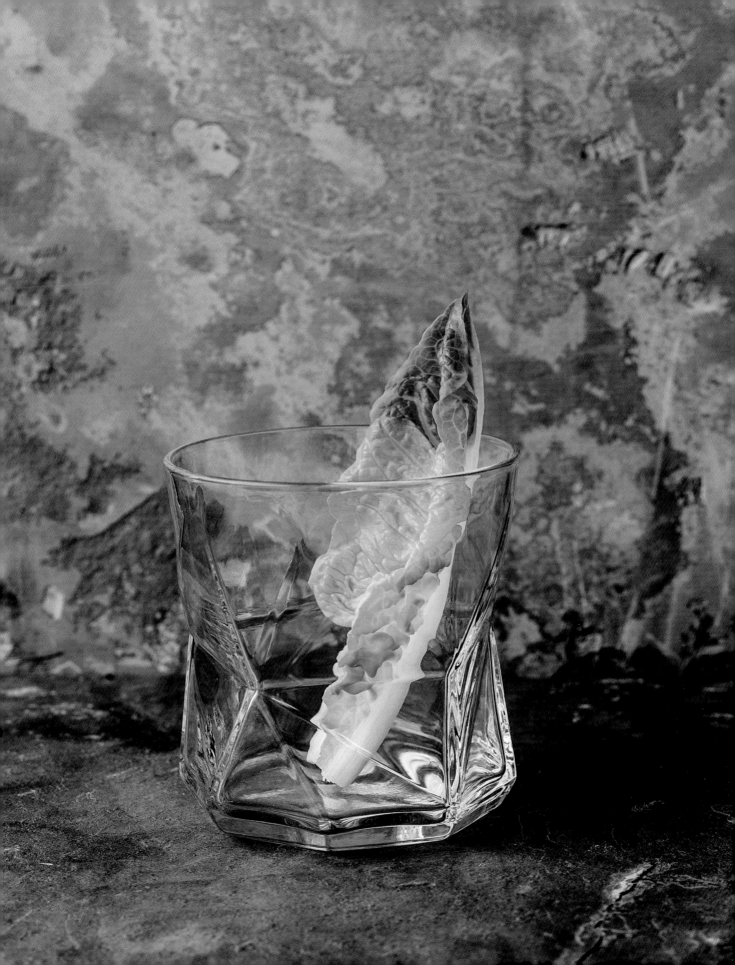

THAI SUNRISE

SERVES 1

Ingredients

1 PEAR

4 FRESH LYCHEES

1 ¾ cups SPINACH

**6 FRESH THAI BASIL LEAVES,
PLUS EXTRA TO GARNISH**

1 cup chilled water

¼-inch **PIECE FRESH GINGER, PEELED**

juice of ½ lime

>SMOOTH<

- PEEL AND CORE THE PEAR AND PEEL AND PIT THE LYCHEES.

- PUT THE SPINACH, BASIL, AND WATER INTO A BLENDER AND BLEND UNTIL SMOOTH.

- ADD THE PEAR, LYCHEES, GINGER, AND LIME JUICE AND BLEND UNTIL SMOOTH. SERVE IMMEDIATELY, GARNISHED WITH A SPRIG OF THAI BASIL.

HAIL THE KALE

SERVES 1

BLEND IT<

Ingredients

½ cup **SHREDDED GREEN
CURLY KALE**

⅔ cup **COCONUT FLESH**

1 ½ cups **CHILLED ALMOND MILK**

1 tablespoon sunflower seeds

¼ teaspoon **GROUND CINNAMON**

- PUT THE KALE, COCONUT, ALMOND MILK, SEEDS, AND CINNAMON INTO A BLENDER.

- BLEND TOGETHER UNTIL SMOOTH AND CREAMY (THIS MIGHT TAKE A LITTLE LONGER THAN USUAL BECAUSE OF THE COCONUT). SERVE IMMEDIATELY.

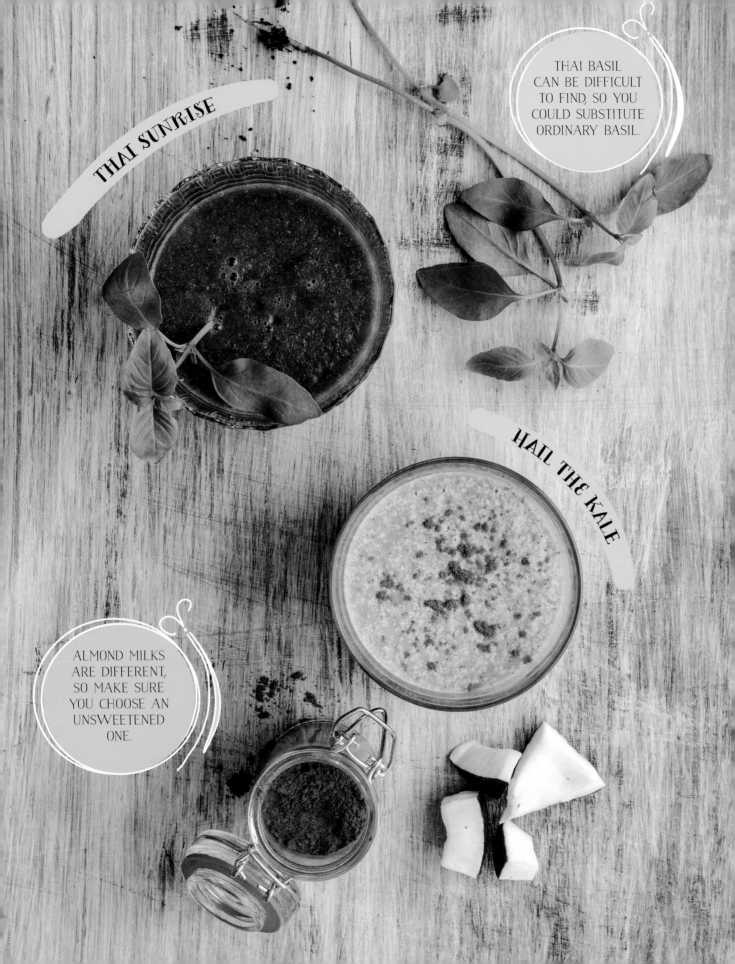

THAI SUNRISE

HAIL THE KALE

THAI BASIL CAN BE DIFFICULT TO FIND, SO YOU COULD SUBSTITUTE ORDINARY BASIL.

ALMOND MILKS ARE DIFFERENT, SO MAKE SURE YOU CHOOSE AN UNSWEETENED ONE.

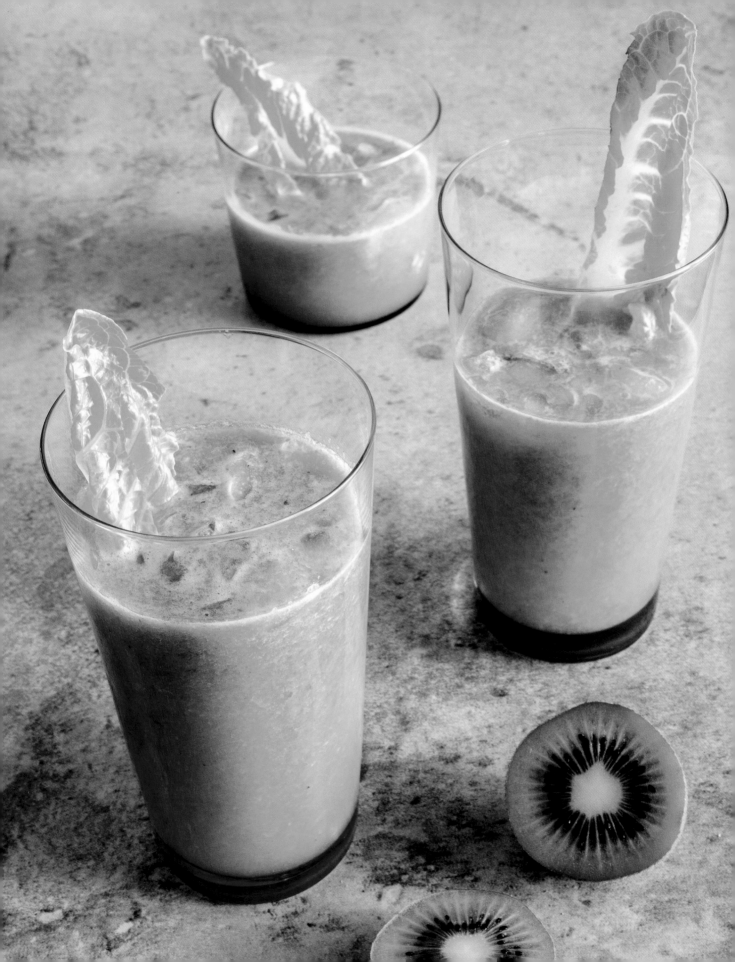

KIWI QUENCHER

A COMBINATION TO GET YOU GLOWING FROM THE INSIDE OUT—JEWEL-LIKE KIWIFRUIT BLENDED WITH JUICY GREEN GRAPES AND THIRST-QUENCHING LETTUCE.

SERVES 1

Ingredients

½ ROMAINE LETTUCE

4 KIWIS, PEELED

¾ CUP GREEN GRAPES

1 LARGE PEAR, HALVED

small handful ice, to serve (optional)

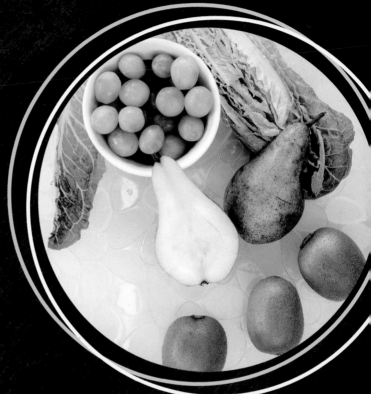

MIX IT UP

- PEEL OFF A LETTUCE LEAF AND RESERVE. FEED THE KIWIS, GRAPES, LETTUCE, AND PEAR THROUGH A JUICER.

- FILL A GLASS HALFWAY WITH ICE, IF USING, THEN POUR IN THE JUICE.

- DECORATE WITH THE RESERVED LETTUCE LEAF AND SERVE IMMEDIATELY.

GREEN GODDESS

GINSENG IS A NATURAL STIMULANT THAT HELPS TO COMBAT STRESS AND LIFTS THE MOOD. THIS JUICE ALSO AIDS LIVER AND KIDNEY FUNCTION AND PREVENTS FLUID RETENTION.

Ingredients

1 GINSENG TEA BAG OR
1 teaspoon GINSENG TEA

2/3 CUP boiling water

1 APPLE, HALVED

1 1/2 CUPS ARUGULA

THE GLORY OF GINSENG

GINSENG IS A SLOW-GROWING PLANT WITH FLESHY ROOTS. AS WELL AS A POWERFUL APHRODISIAC AND TONIC, IT IS ALSO BELIEVED TO ACT AS AN APPETITE SUPPRESSANT, WHICH CAN HELP TO ENCOURAGE WEIGHT LOSS.

TIME FOR TEA

- PUT THE TEA BAG OR TEA INTO A CUP, POUR THE BOILING WATER OVER THE TEA, AND LET STEEP FOR 4 MINUTES.

- STRAIN THE WATER INTO A HEATPROOF GLASS.

- FEED THE APPLE AND ARUGULA THROUGH A JUICER.

- STIR THE JUICE INTO THE TEA AND SERVE WARM OR COLD.

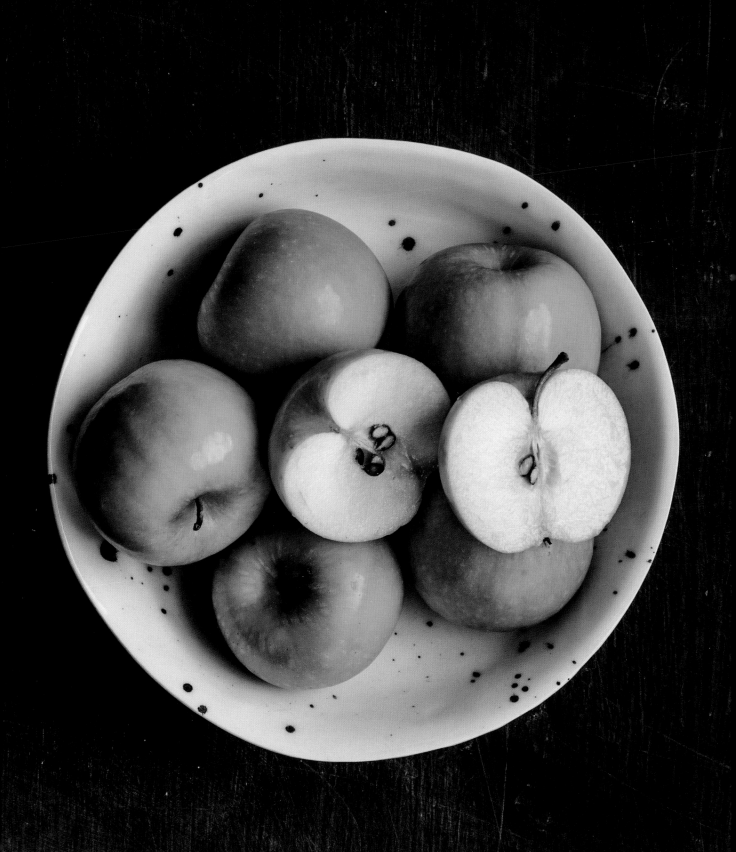

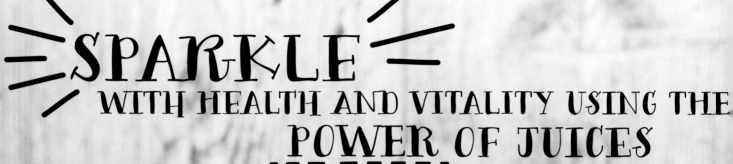

SPARKLE
WITH HEALTH AND VITALITY USING THE
POWER OF JUICES

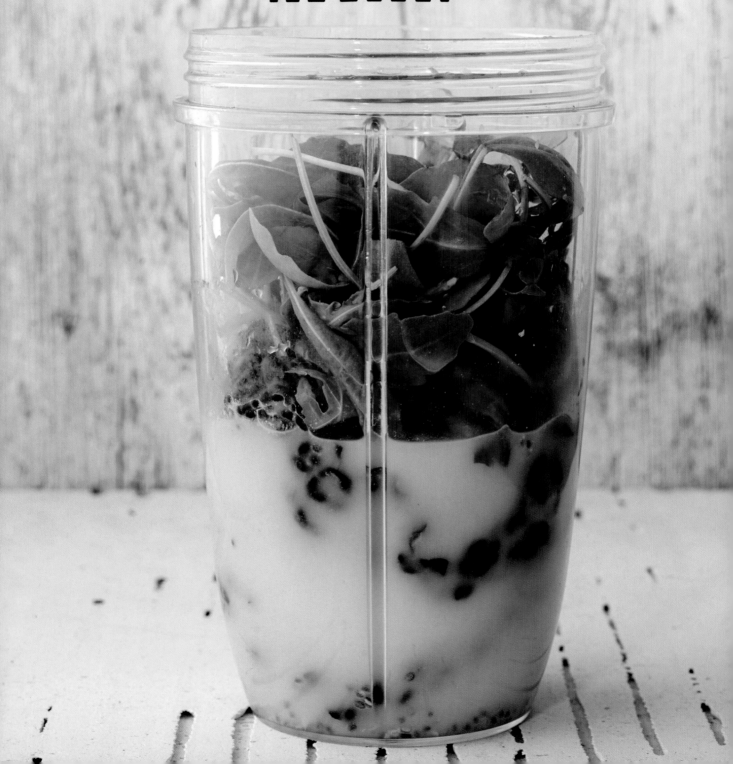

PACKED WITH ALL THE VITAMINS, MINERALS, AND PLANT COMPOUNDS YOU NEED, A DIET RICH IN JUICED OR BLENDED VEGETABLES AND FRUIT CAN MAKE A REAL DIFFERENCE TO HOW YOU LOOK AS WELL AS TO YOUR PHYSICAL WELL-BEING. TAKE A LOOK AT THE BENEFITS!

GREEN FOR YOUR SKIN

Kale (as well as carrots, Swiss chard, spinach, and many other leafy greens) are rich in a pigment called beta-carotene, a powerful antioxidant that helps to slow the aging process of cells to keep your skin looking young and healthy. Kale is also rich in potassium and is a source of anti-inflammatory omega-3 fats, both of which can help reduce acne and other and other skin complaints.

Parsley has high levels of vitamin K, which can improve skin elasticity and speed up the wound-healing process.

Kiwi, bell peppers, and kale are all rich in vitamin C, vital not only for general skin health but also the production of collagen, which maintains skin elasticity and helps prevent wrinkles.

The pith of citrus fruit is rich in bioflavonoids—compounds that help strengthen blood capillaries in the skin and prevent broken veins.

Almonds, Brazil nuts, avocados, and sunflower seeds are rich in vitamin E to combat dry skin and brittle nails, while cacao, pumpkin, and sunflower seeds are great sources of zinc, an antioxidant that keeps skin healthy and disease-free, and helps healing as well as strengthening weak nails.

GREEN FOR YOUR HAIR

For healthy hair and to help prevent hair loss, you can't beat plenty of dark, leafy greens, such as collard greens, cabbage, kale, and broccoli. These contain high amounts of iron—to keep follicles healthy and the scalp in good condition—as well as vitamin C, which helps the body absorb iron. Finally, they are rich in carotenes that are essential for the production of sebum to combat dry hair and give it shine.

GREEN FOR YOUR EYES

To make the whites of your eyes brighter and whiter, all the wonderful vitamin-C-rich juicing fruit and vegetables, such as citrus, leafy greens, kiwi, watercress, and mangoes, are what you need. For good general eye health and if you experience conditions such as dry eye, make sure you get enough zinc and omega-3s—try juices that contain nuts and seeds.

GREEN FOR YOUR TEETH AND GUMS

Soy products, cacao, almonds, Brazil nuts, and leafy greens are great sources of calcium, which is vital for maintaining teeth as well as bones. Alkaline foods, such as greens, avocados, and almonds, can help combat the acidity that can cause tooth enamel to lose mineral density.

To prevent gum disease, get your fill of catechins—found in great amounts in green tea, cacao, and raw, unpeeled apples. And drink your spinach—it is one of the few rich vegetable sources of coenzyme Q10, a compound that keeps gums healthy and free from bleeding.

GREEN FOR YOUR WELL-BEING

It's proven that a diet high in fresh vegetables, fruit, and other plant foods and extracts is linked to protection from the major diseases, such as cancer, diabetes, and cardiovascular disease. If you choose a range of juices, blended drinks, and soups from this book and have them regularly, you will benefit not only from this protective effect but you will, almost certainly, find that your general health and well-being improve. From all the small benefits listed above to improvements, such as greater energy, better sleep, and mood, the positives you'll get from going green and clean are huge.

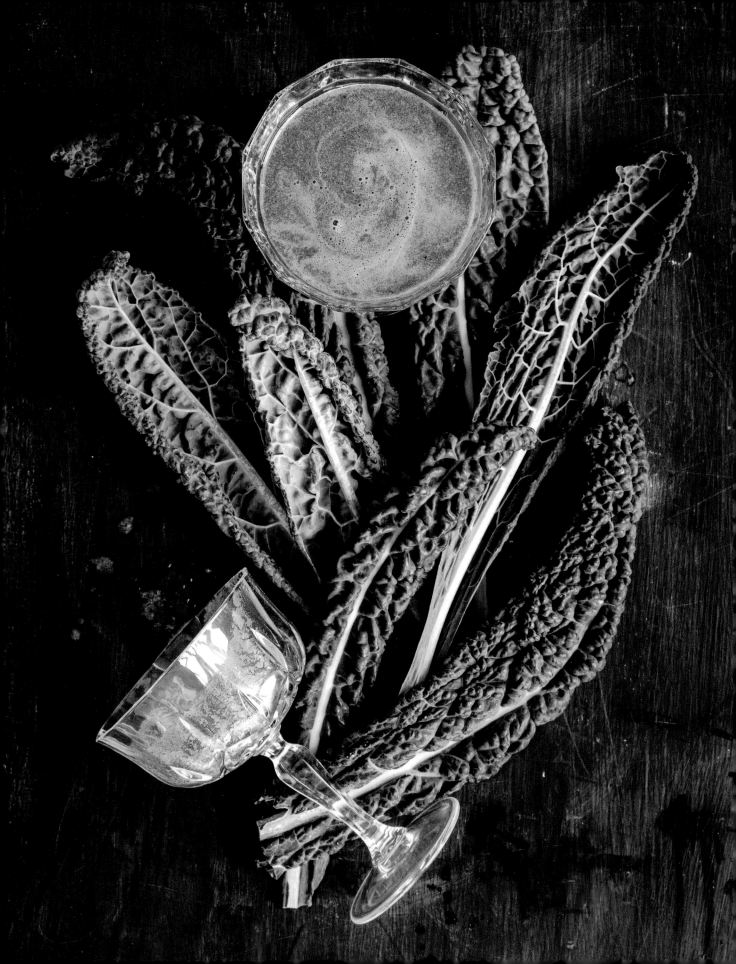

GREEN & MEAN

INSPIRED BY THE ITALIAN *CAVOLO NERO*, WHICH TRANSLATES AS "BLACK CABBAGE," THIS JUICE USES TUSCAN KALE. IT IS LOADED WITH VITAMINS, MINERALS, AND IRON, AND IS THE HERO OF THIS JUICE.

SERVES 1

Ingredients

2 CARROTS

1¼ CUPS TUSCAN KALE (when chopped)

½ CUP TURNIP GREENS (when chopped)

1⅓ CUPS GREEN GRAPES

¼ CUP FRESH FLAT-LEAF PARSLEY

IF YOU CAN'T GET YOUR HANDS ON TUSCAN KALE, USE ANOTHER DARK-LEAFED KALE INSTEAD.

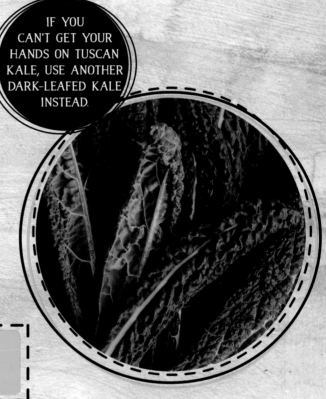

GET JUICING

- COARSELY CHOP THE CARROTS, TUSCAN KALE, AND TURNIP GREENS JUST ENOUGH TO FEED THROUGH THE JUICER.

- FEED THE GRAPES, PARSLEY, CARROTS, TUSCAN KALE, AND TURNIP GREENS INTO THE FUNNEL OF A JUICER AND JUICE.

- STIR WELL AND SERVE IMMEDIATELY.

SPROUT TONIC

BRUSSELS SPROUTS MIGHT SEEM LIKE A
WINTER DINNER STAPLE, BUT DRINKING THEM
IN A SMOOTHIE LIKE THIS MEANS YOU CAN EAT
YOUR GREENS ALL YEAR ROUND.

SERVES 1

Ingredients

4 BRUSSELS SPROUTS

¾ CUP CHOPPED BEET GREENS

½ CUP CHOPPED SWISS CHARD

1 CUP unsweetened rice milk

THE RICE
MILK CAN BE
REPLACED WITH
ALMOND OR
COCONUT MILK.

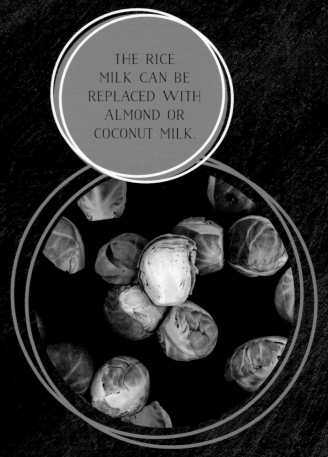

BLEND IT

- PUT THE BRUSSELS SPROUTS, BEET GREENS, AND SWISS CHARD
  INTO A BLENDER.

- POUR IN THE RICE MILK AND BLEND UNTIL SMOOTH AND
  CREAMY. SERVE IMMEDIATELY.

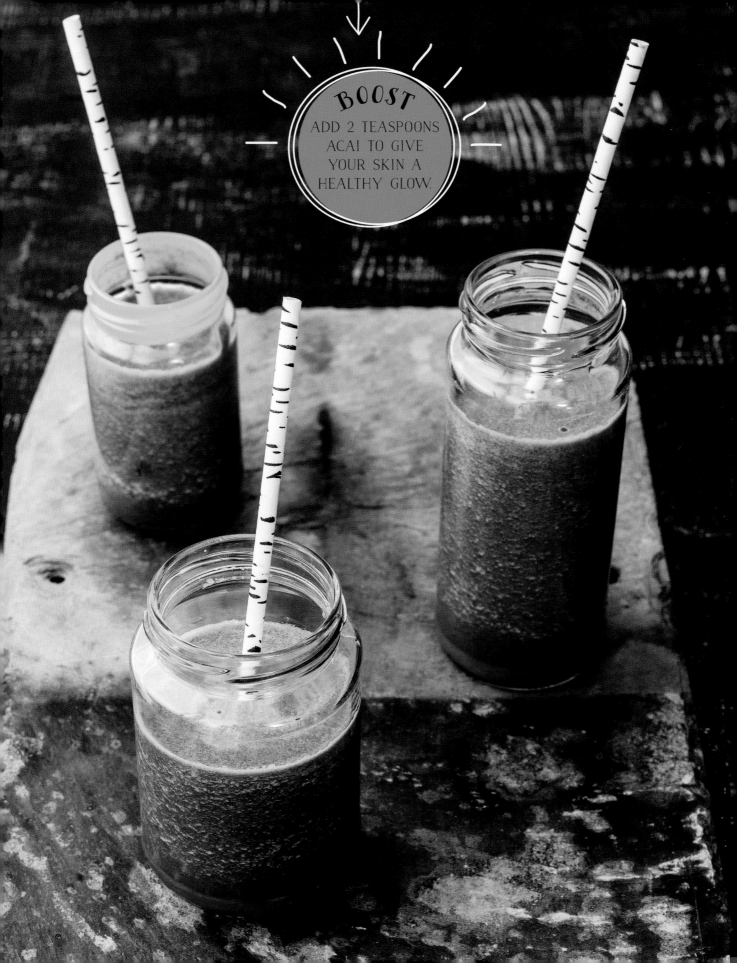

BOOST

ADD 2 TEASPOONS
ACAI TO GIVE
YOUR SKIN A
HEALTHY GLOW.

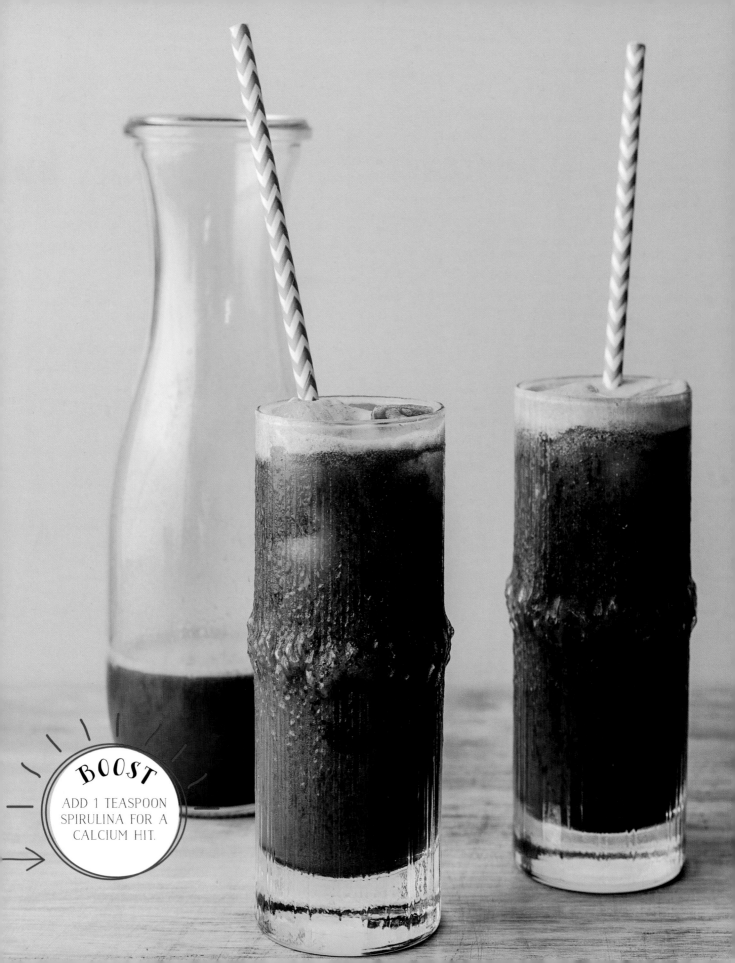

BOOST

ADD 1 TEASPOON
SPIRULINA FOR A
CALCIUM HIT.

BEET IT!

SERVES 1

EARTHY AND SWEET, BEETS BRING A LOT
TO THE TABLE. THE LEAVES SHOULD NOT BE
DISCARDED—THEY CAN BE ENJOYED PREPARED
IN THE SAME WAY AS SPINACH.

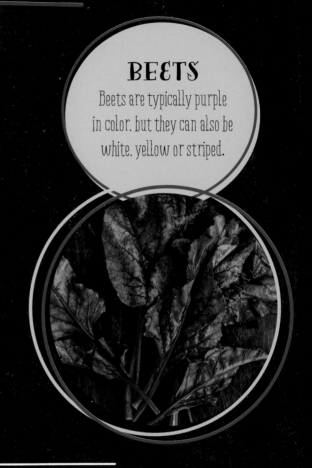

BEETS
Beets are typically purple
in color, but they can also be
white, yellow or striped.

Ingredients

1 BEET

1 GREEN APPLE

1 1/2 CUPS ARUGULA

1 HEAD OF RADICCHIO

1 CUP BEET GREENS

> READY, STEADY ... JUICE!

- COARSELY CHOP THE BEET AND APPLE.

- FEED THE ARUGULA, RADICCHIO, BEET GREENS, APPLE,
  AND BEET INTO THE JUICER FUNNEL AND JUICE.

- STIR WELL AND SERVE IMMEDIATELY.

MANGO & LIME BONE BUILDER

SERVES 1

THIS PRETTY, GREEN-SPECKLED DRINK LOOKS MANGO-FREE, BUT THE FRUIT'S NATURAL SWEETNESS PERFECTLY BALANCES THE KALE.

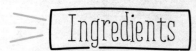

Ingredients

1 tablespoon SESAME SEEDS

juice of ½ lime

½ cup SHREDDED GREEN CURLY KALE

1 MANGO, PEELED, PITTED, AND COARSELY CHOPPED

1 cup unsweetened rice, almond, or soy milk

small handful crushed ice

> WHIZZ IT!

- PUT THE SESAME SEEDS INTO A BLENDER AND BLEND UNTIL FINELY GROUND.

- ADD THE LIME JUICE, KALE, AND MANGO AND BLEND UNTIL WELL COMBINED.

- ADD THE MILK AND CRUSHED ICE AND BLEND AGAIN UNTIL SMOOTH. POUR INTO A GLASS AND SERVE IMMEDIATELY.

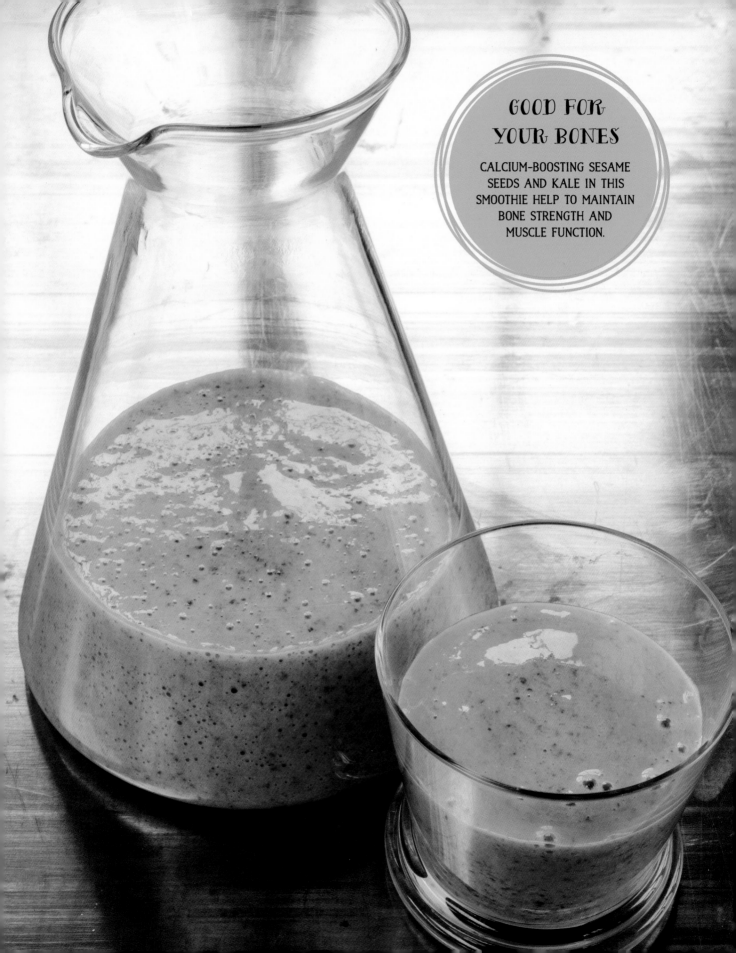

PEAR & LEMON WAKE-UP CALL

SERVES 1

JUICY SHOTS SUCH AS THIS ZINGY MOUTHFUL ARE PERFECT FOR A QUICK ENERGY HIT.

Ingredients

¼ FENNEL BULB

¼ PEAR, PEELED AND CORED

1-inch PIECE FRESH GINGER, PEELED

juice of ½ lemon

2½ tablespoons chilled water

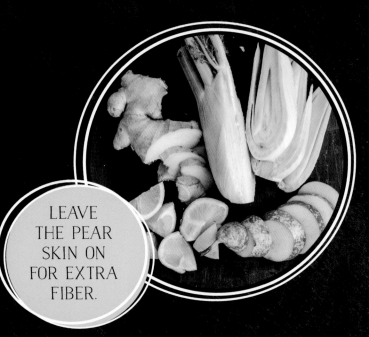

LEAVE THE PEAR SKIN ON FOR EXTRA FIBER.

GIVE IT A WHIRL

- SLICE THE FENNEL AND PUT IT INTO A BLENDER. ADD THE PEAR TO THE BLENDER WITH THE GINGER AND LEMON JUICE.

- POUR IN THE WATER AND BLEND UNTIL SMOOTH. SERVE IMMEDIATELY.

GARDEN CHARGER

DENSE WITH LEAFY GREENS, THIS FRESH AND MINTY
SHOT IS A GREAT WAY TO START YOUR DAY.

SERVES 1

KALE
IS ALWAYS
A GREAT
SUBSTITUTE FOR
SPINACH.

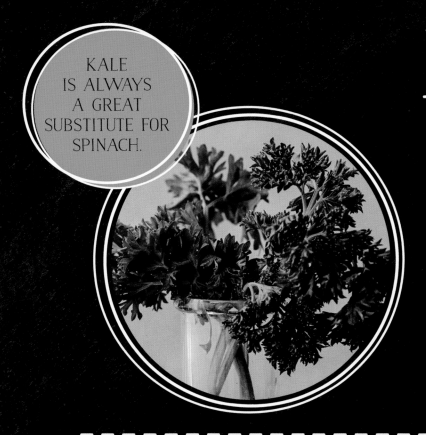

Ingredients
>—<

½ CUP SPINACH

6 FRESH MINT LEAVES

1 teaspoon CHOPPED
FRESH PARSLEY

juice of ½ lime

5 tablespoons chilled water

READY, STEADY ... BLEND!

- PUT THE SPINACH, MINT, PARSLEY, AND LIME JUICE
  INTO A BLENDER.

- POUR IN THE WATER AND BLEND UNTIL SMOOTH.
  SERVE IMMEDIATELY.

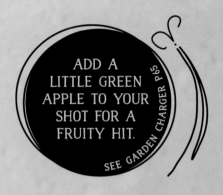

ADD A
LITTLE GREEN
APPLE TO YOUR
SHOT FOR A
FRUITY HIT.

SEE GARDEN CHARGER P65

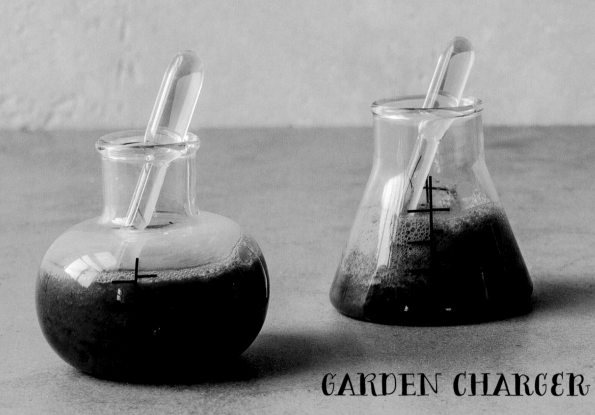

GARDEN CHARGER

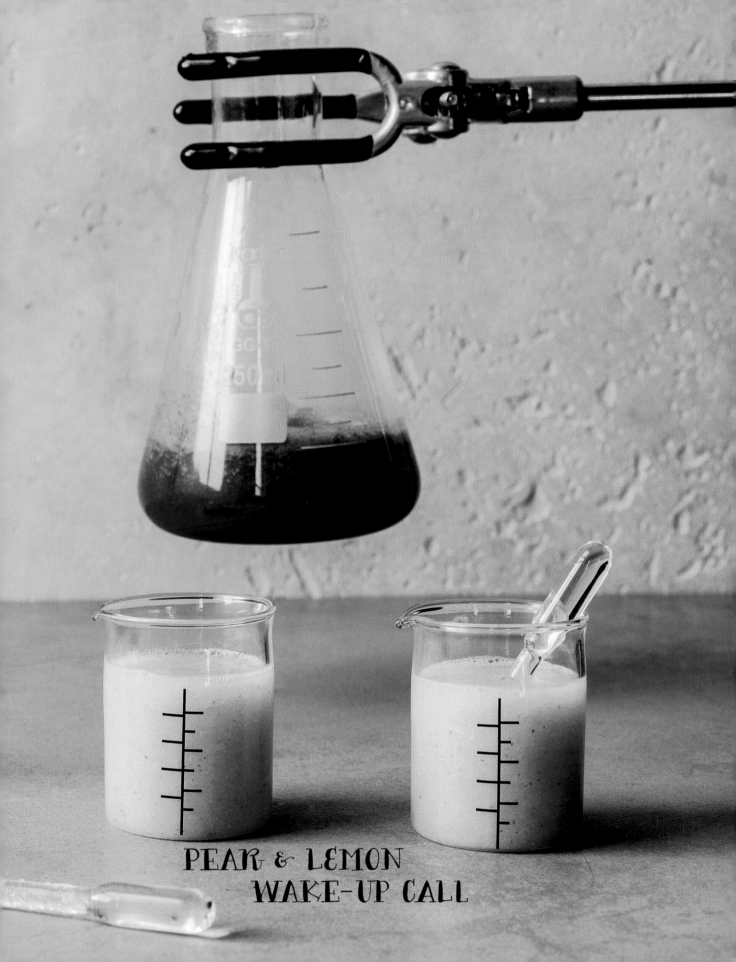

PEAR & LEMON
WAKE-UP CALL

ROCKET FUEL SOUP

THE MILD SPICE FROM THE ARUGULA AND MUSTARD GREENS IS SOFTENED BY THE AVOCADO AND COCONUT MILK, CREATING A CREAMY BUT HEALTHY SOUP.

SERVES 1

Ingredients

¾ CUP ARUGULA, PLUS EXTRA TO GARNISH

⅓ CUP MUSTARD GREENS

1 CUP chilled water

½ AVOCADO, PITTED AND FLESH SCOOPED FROM SKIN

½ CUP coconut milk

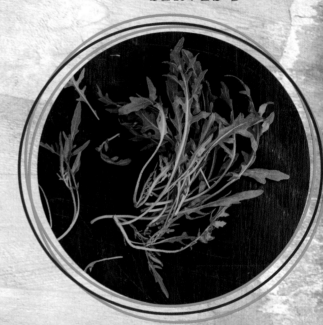

GET BLENDING

- PUT THE ARUGULA, MUSTARD GREENS, AND WATER INTO A BLENDER AND BLEND UNTIL SMOOTH.

- ADD THE AVOCADO TO THE BLENDER WITH THE COCONUT MILK AND BLEND UNTIL SMOOTH AND CREAMY.

- SERVE IMMEDIATELY OR CHILL IN THE REFRIGERATOR. STIR WELL JUST BEFORE SERVING, GARNISHED WITH A FEW ARUGULA LEAVES.

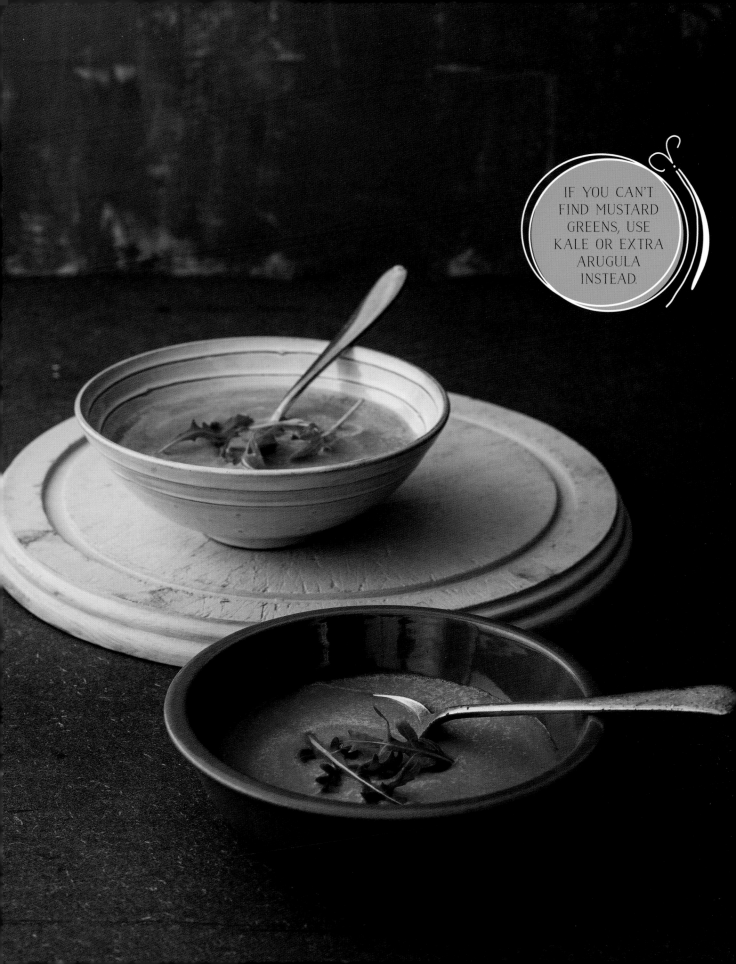

IF YOU CAN'T
FIND MUSTARD
GREENS, USE
KALE OR EXTRA
ARUGULA
INSTEAD.

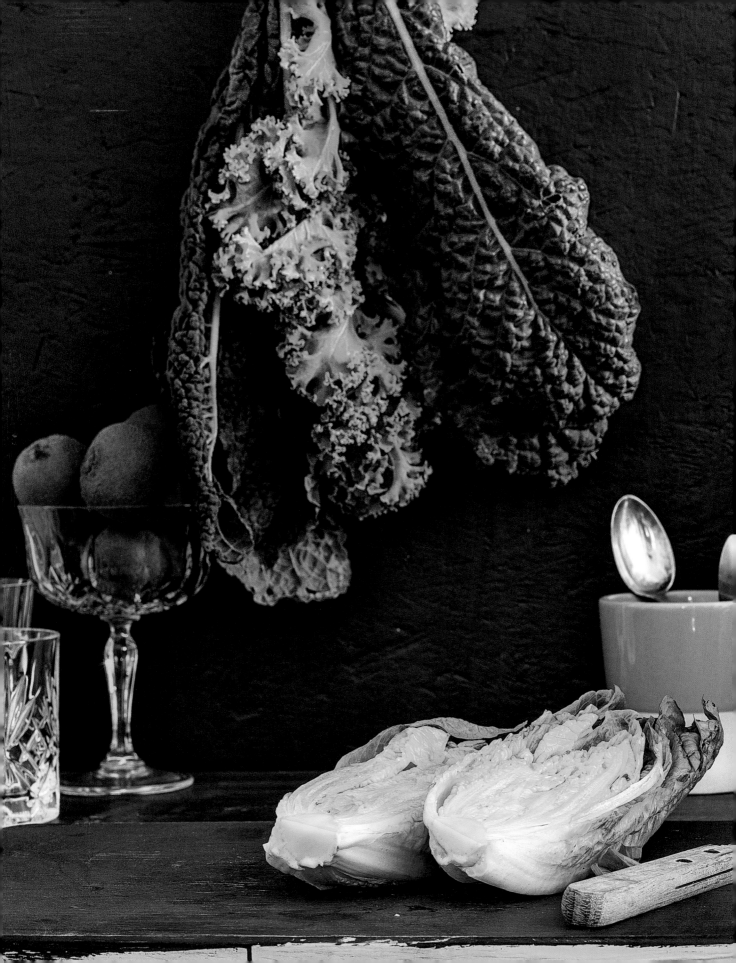

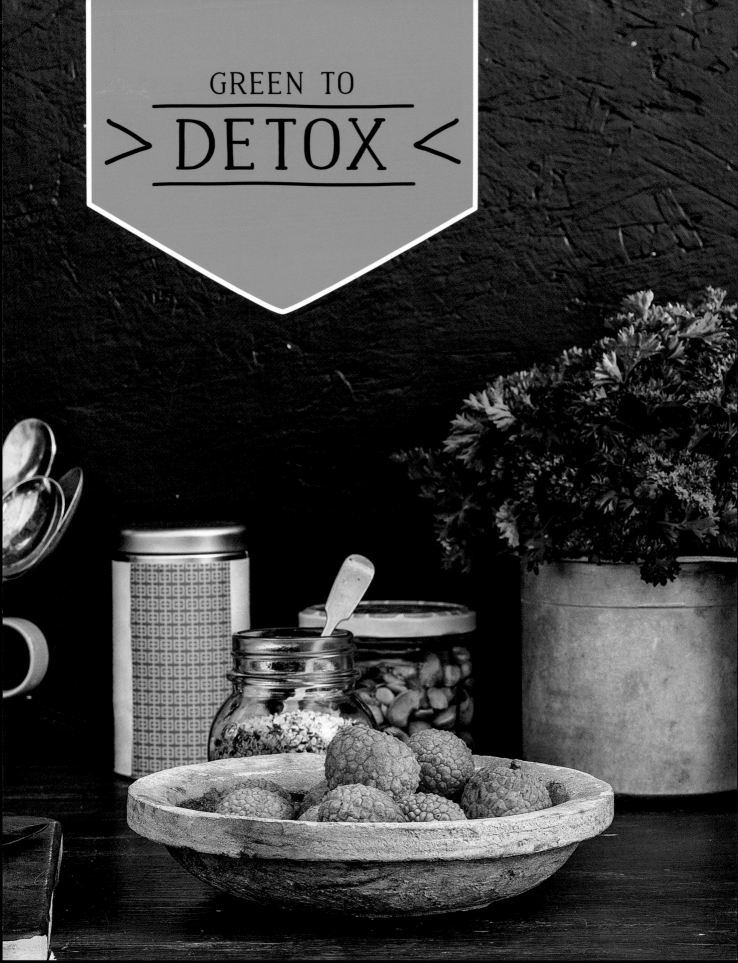

GREEN TO
> DETOX <

GREEN COLADA

FLAXSEED ARE BELIEVED TO HELP FORTIFY THE
SKIN'S BARRIERS AND ARE A SIMPLE ADDITION
TO THIS COOLING JUICE.

SERVES 1

Ingredients

3 ½ cups SPINACH

⅓ CUCUMBER

½ cup FRESH MINT

1 cup coconut milk

½ teaspoon flaxseed

1 teaspoon CHLOROPHYLL POWDER

crushed ice, to serve (optional)

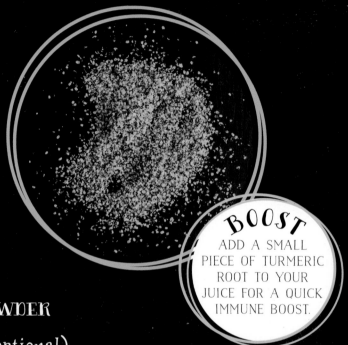

BOOST
ADD A SMALL
PIECE OF TURMERIC
ROOT TO YOUR
JUICE FOR A QUICK
IMMUNE BOOST.

> TRY THIS JUICE

- COARSELY CHOP THE SPINACH AND CUCUMBER, THEN FEED
  INTO THE JUICER FUNNEL WITH THE MINT AND JUICE.

- STIR IN THE COCONUT MILK, FLAXSEED, AND
  CHLOROPHYLL POWDER UNTIL COMBINED. TO SERVE, FILL
  A GLASS WITH CRUSHED ICE AND POUR IN THE JUICE.

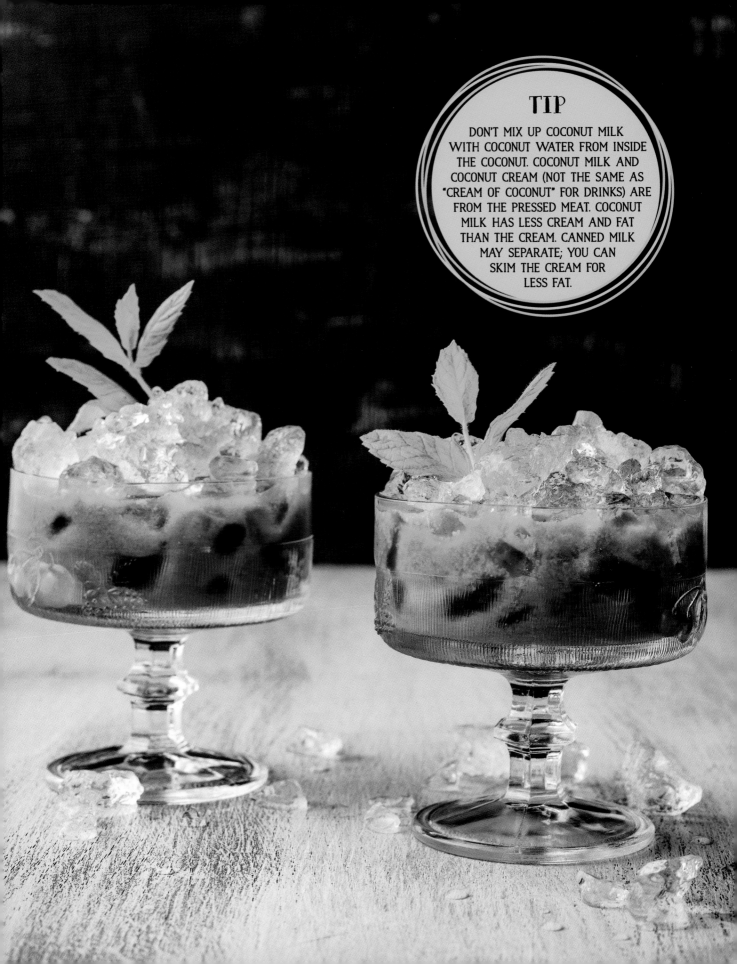

TIP

DON'T MIX UP COCONUT MILK WITH COCONUT WATER FROM INSIDE THE COCONUT. COCONUT MILK AND COCONUT CREAM (NOT THE SAME AS "CREAM OF COCONUT" FOR DRINKS) ARE FROM THE PRESSED MEAT. COCONUT MILK HAS LESS CREAM AND FAT THAN THE CREAM. CANNED MILK MAY SEPARATE; YOU CAN SKIM THE CREAM FOR LESS FAT.

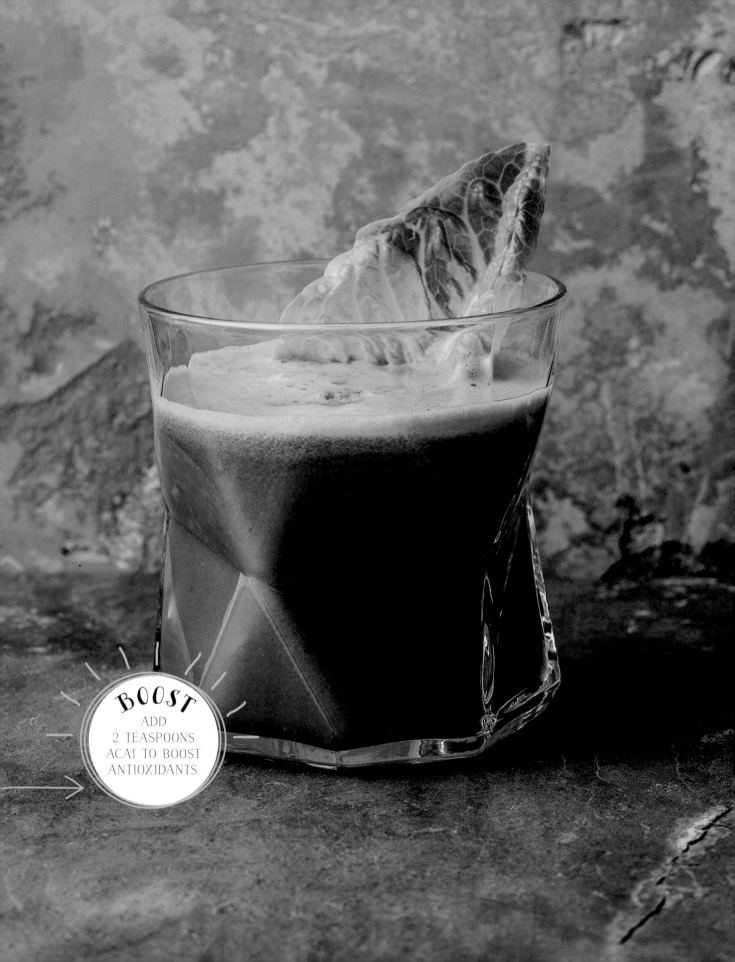

BOOST ADD 2 TEASPOONS ACAI TO BOOST ANTIOXIDANTS.

LETTUCE ELIXIR

SERVES 1

LETTUCE, CELERY, AND APPLE ALL CONTAIN A LOT OF WATER, WHICH IS ESSENTIAL FOR THE BODY TO BE ABLE TO FLUSH OUT TOXINS.

Ingredients

⅙ ROMAINE LETTUCE, PLUS EXTRA TO GARNISH

4 CELERY STALKS

1 GREEN APPLE

½ CUP FRESH FLAT-LEAF PARSLEY

1 teaspoon spirulina powder

crushed ice, to serve (optional)

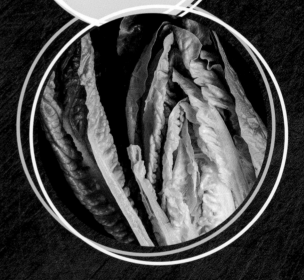

NOT ALL LETTUCES ARE CREATED EQUAL. ROMAINE LETTUCE HAS ONE OF THE HIGHEST NUTRITIONAL VALUES OF ALL, SO CHOOSE IT OVER OTHER VARIETIES.

JUICE IT UP

- COARSELY CHOP THE LETTUCE, CELERY, AND APPLE, THEN FEED THEM INTO THE FUNNEL OF A JUICER WITH THE PARSLEY AND JUICE.

- STIR IN THE SPIRULINA POWDER UNTIL COMBINED.

- POUR OVER CRUSHED ICE, IF USING, AND SERVE IMMEDIATELY, GARNISHED WITH A SMALL LETTUCE LEAF.

GRAPE & LYCHEE REVIVER

SERVES 1

GO ASIAN WITH FRAGRANT LYCHEES, THOUGHT BY THE CHINESE TO BE THE SYMBOL OF LOVE. BLEND THEM WITH CREAMY, SMOOTH AVOCADO AND NATURALLY SWEET GRAPES FOR THE PERFECT PICK-ME-UP TO REHYDRATE AND FIGHT FATIGUE.

Ingredients

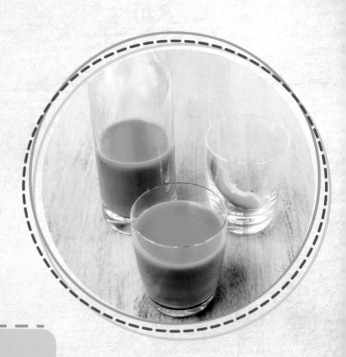

2 cups GREEN GRAPES

2 cups YOUNG SPINACH

$\frac{1}{2}$ RIPE AVOCADO, PITTED AND FLESH SCOOPED FROM THE SKIN, PLUS A SLICE TO SERVE (OPTIONAL)

5 LYCHEES, PEELED AND PITTED

small handful crushed ice

$\frac{1}{2}$ cup chilled water

BLEND IT!

- FEED THE GRAPES AND SPINACH INTO A JUICER FUNNEL, AND JUICE.

- POUR THE JUICE INTO A BLENDER, ADD THE AVOCADO, LYCHEES, AND CRUSHED ICE, AND BLEND UNTIL SMOOTH.

- ADD THE WATER AND BLEND AGAIN. POUR INTO A GLASS, ADD THE AVOCADO SLICE, IF USING, AND SERVE IMMEDIATELY.

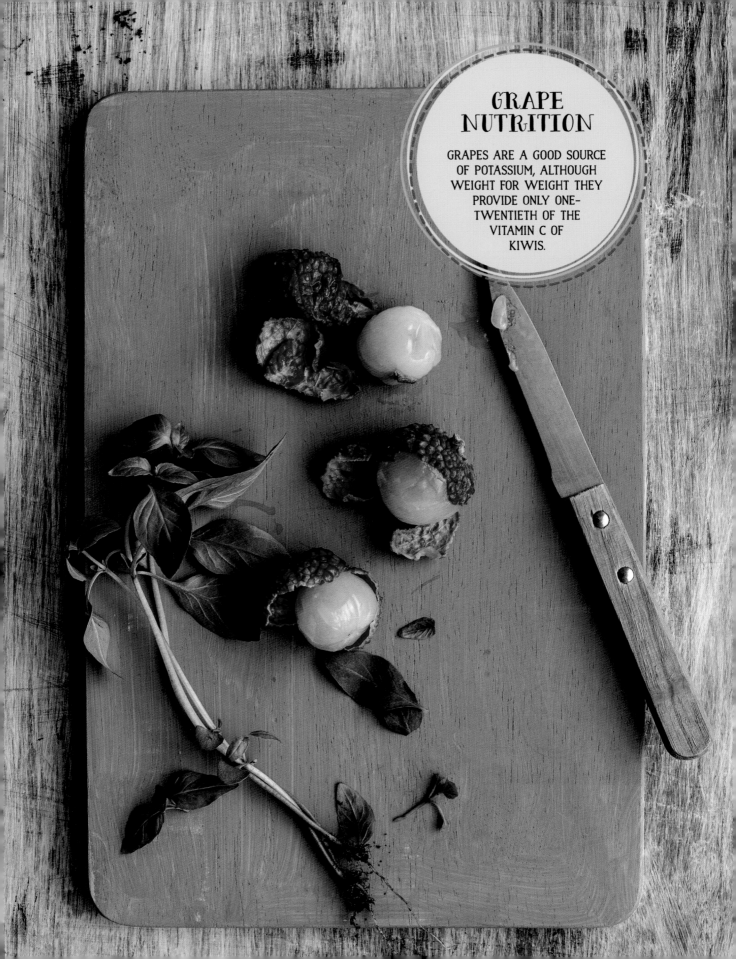

GRAPE NUTRITION

GRAPES ARE A GOOD SOURCE OF POTASSIUM, ALTHOUGH WEIGHT FOR WEIGHT THEY PROVIDE ONLY ONE-TWENTIETH OF THE VITAMIN C OF KIWIS.

MOTHER EARTH

Ingredients

½ cup CURLY GREEN KALE

1½ cups chilled water

2 CELERY STALKS

½ AVOCADO, PITTED AND FLESH SCOOPED FROM SKIN

1 SMALL PIECE TURMERIC ROOT, PEELED

1 tablespoon YUZU JUICE

1-inch PIECE FRESH GINGER, PEELED

1 teaspoon bee pollen

1 tablespoon goji berries

>BLEND<

- SHRED THE KALE, PUT INTO A BLENDER WITH THE WATER, AND BLEND UNTIL SMOOTH.

- CHOP THE CELERY AND AVOCADO AND ADD TO THE BLENDER WITH THE TURMERIC, YUZU JUICE, GINGER, BEE POLLEN, AND GOJI BERRIES. BLEND UNTIL SMOOTH AND SERVE IMMEDIATELY.

COCONUT RESTORER

SERVES 1

Ingredients

½ cup SHREDDED TUSCAN KALE

½ cup CHOPPED BEET GREENS

1 teaspoon CHIA SEEDS, PLUS A PINCH TO GARNISH

2 teaspoons ALMOND BUTTER

1 cup coconut milk

½ cup chilled water

MIX IT<

- ADD THE SHREDDED TUSCAN KALE TO A BLENDER WITH THE BEET GREENS, CHIA SEEDS, AND ALMOND BUTTER.

- POUR IN THE COCONUT MILK AND WATER, AND BLEND UNTIL SMOOTH AND CREAMY. SERVE IMMEDIATELY, SPRINKLED WITH CHIA SEEDS TO GARNISH.

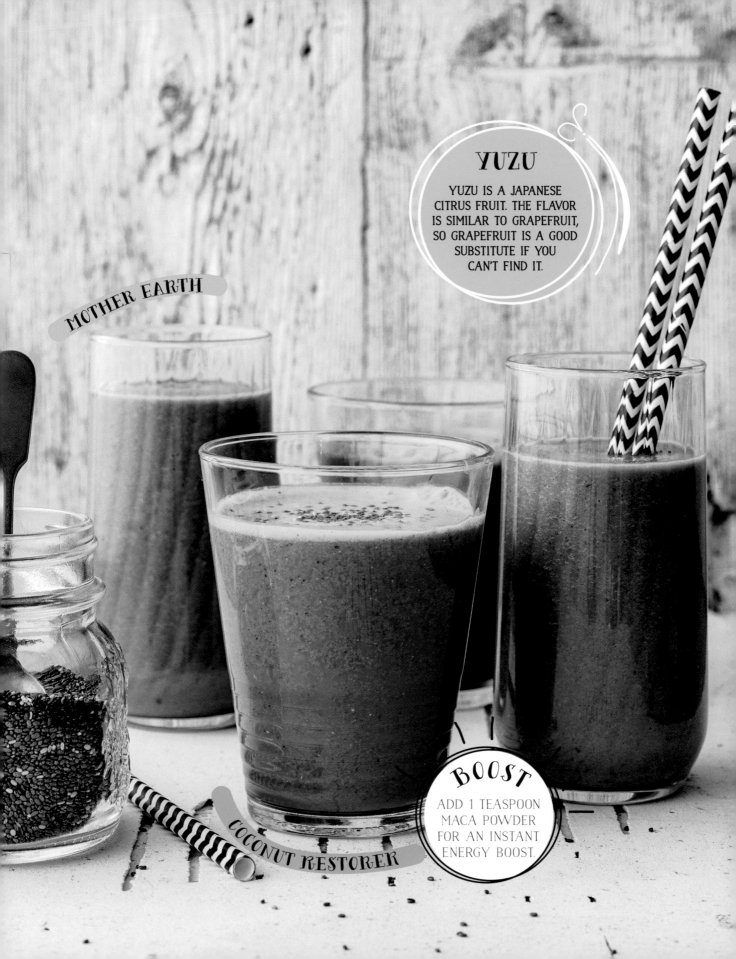

YUZU

YUZU IS A JAPANESE CITRUS FRUIT. THE FLAVOR IS SIMILAR TO GRAPEFRUIT, SO GRAPEFRUIT IS A GOOD SUBSTITUTE IF YOU CAN'T FIND IT.

MOTHER EARTH

COCONUT RESTORER

BOOST

ADD 1 TEASPOON MACA POWDER FOR AN INSTANT ENERGY BOOST.

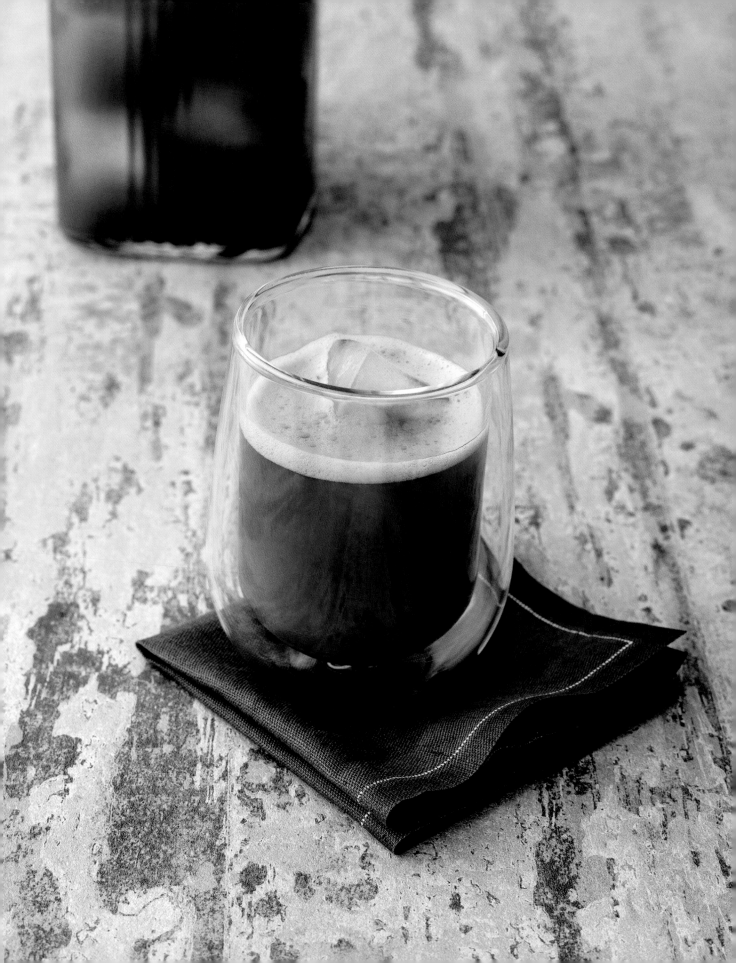

GREEN TEA PUNCH

SERVES 1

GREEN TEA IS PACKED WITH ANTIOXIDANTS. COMBINED WITH GINSENG AND WHEATGRASS, THIS IS A GREAT DETOXIFYING JUICE THAT WILL CLEANSE YOU FROM THE INSIDE OUT.

>Ingredients<

1½ cups green tea

juice of ½ lemon

¼ teaspoon liquid ginseng

1 teaspoon pea protein

1 teaspoon wheatgrass powder

1 teaspoon maca powder

ice cubes, to serve

MAKE IT A PARTY

SCALE UP THE RECIPE AND CHILL THE PUNCH TO ENJOY WITH FRIENDS ON A HOT DAY.

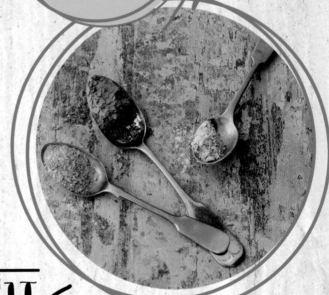

>PACK A PUNCH<

- WHISK THE GREEN TEA WITH THE LEMON JUICE, GINSENG, PEA PROTEIN, WHEATGRASS POWDER, AND MACA POWDER. ALTERNATIVELY, YOU COULD COMBINE THE INGREDIENTS IN A BLENDER.

- SERVE IMMEDIATELY OVER ICE.

MINT REJUVENATOR

SERVES 1

THIS COOLING, CLEANSING DRINK IS GOOD FOR LIVER AND KIDNEY FUNCTION, HELPS LOWER CHOLESTEROL AND RELIEVES TENSION AND INSOMNIA.

Ingredients

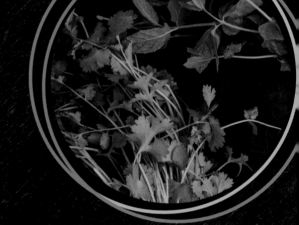

½ HONEYDEW MELON, PEELED AND THICKLY SLICED

3 CUPS YOUNG SPINACH

2 SPRIGS FRESH FLAT-LEAF PARSLEY

3 LARGE STEMS FRESH MINT

small handful ice (optional)

GIVE IT A WHIRL

- FEED THE MELON, SPINACH, PARSLEY, AND TWO STEMS OF MINT THROUGH A JUICER.

- FILL A GLASS HALFWAY WITH ICE, IF USING, THEN POUR IN THE JUICE. GARNISH WITH THE REMAINING STEM OF MINT AND SERVE IMMEDIATELY.

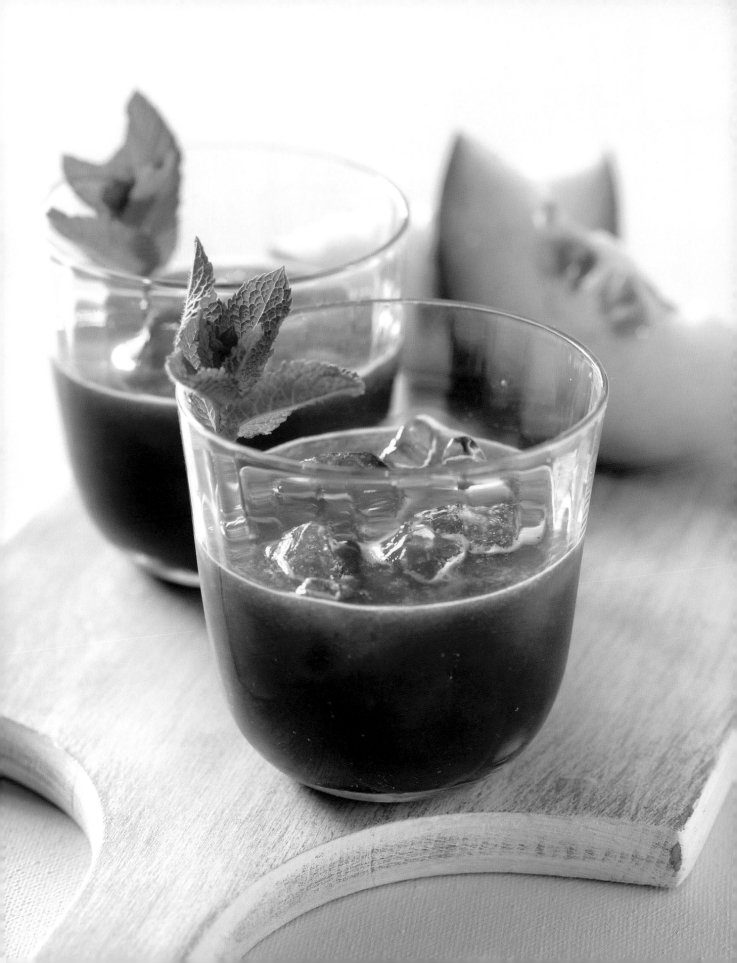

NUTRIENT BOOSTERS

— BIG NEWS FOR YOUR HEALTH

SOMETIMES, LITTLE THINGS MAKE A GOOD DEAL OF DIFFERENCE, AND THAT'S CERTAINLY TRUE IN THE CASE OF NUTRIENT BOOSTERS. THESE ARE NATURAL FOODS THAT, EVEN IN SMALL AMOUNTS, GIVE YOUR HEALTH A SUPERCHARGE. WE'VE PACKED OUR GREEN JUICES WITH THESE SPECIAL INGREDIENTS—LEARN MORE ABOUT THEM HERE.

ACAI

Acai berry is a dark purple fruit that grows on palm trees in the rain forests of South America. Acai has more than double the antioxidants of blueberries, and these compounds can lower the risk of several diseases, including cardiovascular disease and cancer. The berries are also packed with amino acids (protein components), fiber, essential fatty acids, and vitamin C.

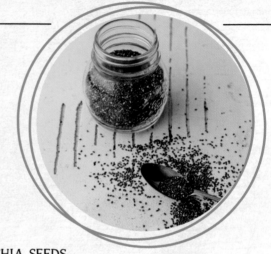

ALOE VERA

Aloe vera is one of the few plant sources of vitamin B12, so it is helpful for vegans. For centuries, it has been used in herbal medicine to calm the digestive tract. It can help irritable bowel syndrome (IBS) and digestive disorders.

BARLEY GRASS

Like wheatgrass, barley grass is rich in immune-boosting, anti-inflammatory chlorophyll (*see page* 25) and can be used fresh or dried.

BEE POLLEN

There is much anecdotal evidence that bee pollen can boost energy and curb food cravings. It also contains vitamin B12 (*see* aloe vera) and rutin, said to prevent blood clots and protect against high blood sugar.

CACAO

Rich in antioxidant plant compounds called polyphenols, cacao is purported by scientists to help prevent heart disease, cancers, and premature aging. However, commercial cocoa powders usually have the flavonoids removed, so choose raw cacao powder.

CHIA SEEDS

Tiny chia seeds are a concentrated source of nutrition, containing healthy omega-3 fatty acids, carbohydrates, protein, fiber, antioxidants, and calcium. Adding the seeds to extracted juices brings down the glycemic index of the drink and helps you feel full for longer.

FLAXSEED, GROUND

Flaxseed (also called linseed) are one of our best nonanimal sources of the essential omega-3 fat alpha-linolenic acid (ALA), which has a range of health benefits. ALA has been shown to reduce inflammation and may help prevent arthritis and heart attacks and reduce high blood pressure.

GINSENG

One of the most used herbal medicines in the world, ginseng has been shown to boost the immune system and lower blood sugar. It's long been used to help give us more energy and stamina, and to improve mood. There are various types of ginseng—the Asian panax ginseng is the one that has been most researched.

GOJI BERRIES

There is some research to show that regularly eating goji berries can protect against heart disease and cancer, as well as boosting immunity and brain activity. The little red berries are rich in carotenes, which boost the immune system and skin health, and help protect your eyesight.

HEMP SEEDS

Hemp seeds and oil are one of the richest sources of ALA (*see* flaxseed). They also contain plant sterols, which help lower blood cholesterol and reduce the risk of heart attacks, as well as being a superb source of vitamin E, which is immune-boosting and known to help keep arteries and skin healthy, and of magnesium for heart and bone health.

MACA

The root of the Peruvian maca plant has a long record of use in traditional medicine. It's said that maca powder can boost energy levels and improve athletic performance, improve mood, and reduce stress levels, as well as support the adrenal glands. The root has also been linked with improvement in menopausal symptoms, including hot flashes.

MANUKA HONEY

A component of New Zealand manuka honey, methylglyoxal (MG), has been shown to have antibiotic qualities. There is a scale for rating the potency of the honey, UMF or unique manuka factor, and a rating of 10 or more is considered a therapeutic level.

SPICES

Spices such as ginger, chile, turmeric, and cinnamon, each have potent effects in promoting good health, even when used in small amounts. Ginger is good for nausea, flatulence, stomach upset, morning sickness, and motion sickness, while turmeric has anti-inflammatory benefits.

SPIRULINA

Spirulina is an alkaline, blue-green algae similar to chlorella (*see page* 25). It is antiviral, has beneficial effects on the digestive system and bowel, and is also anti-inflammatory, so it can help protect us against certain diseases, such as rheumatoid arthritis.

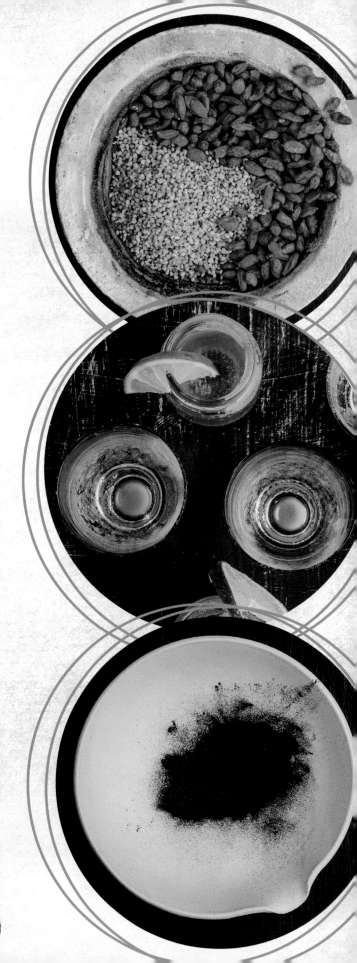

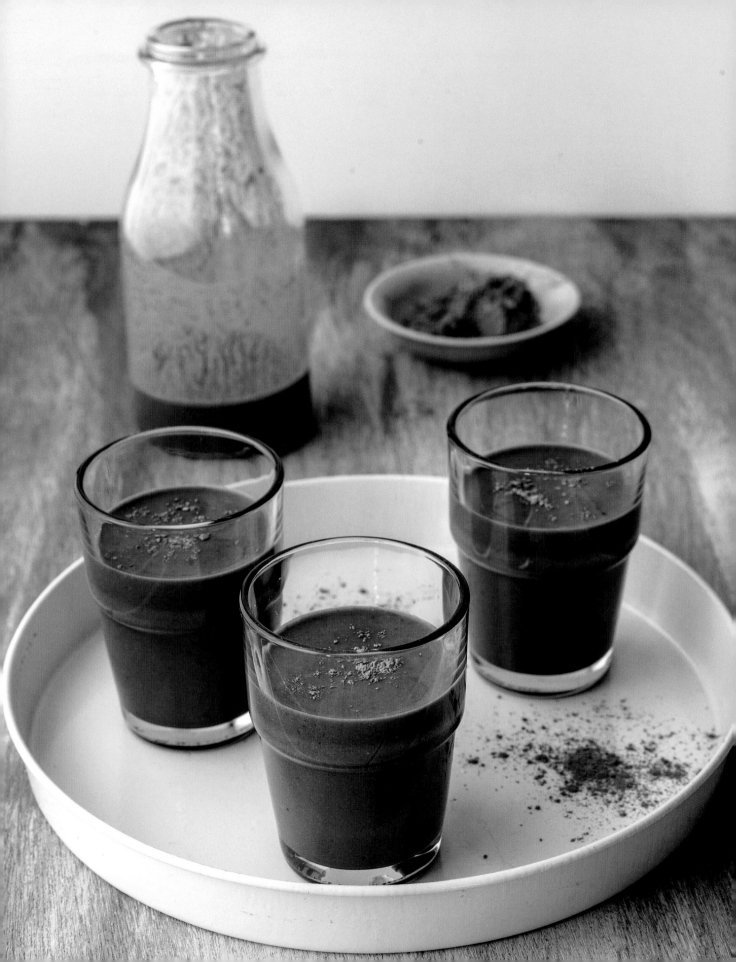

COCO BOMB

THIS CREAMY SMOOTHIE TASTES LIKE A DECADENT TREAT BUT IS ACTUALLY GOOD FOR YOU!

Ingredients

2/3 CUP CHOPPED CURLY GREEN KALE

1 CUP chilled water

1 teaspoon hemp seeds
or hemp seed oil

1 SMALL FROZEN BANANA

1 teaspoon RAW CACAO POWDER, PLUS A SMALL PINCH TO GARNISH

1/4 VANILLA BEAN, SEEDS SCRAPED

TIP
TO FREEZE BANANAS, PEEL THEM, THEN FREEZE THEM ON A TRAY FOR 30 MINUTES, SPACED WELL APART. WHEN FROZEN, TRANSFER TO PLASTIC FOOD BAGS OR PLASTIC CONTAINERS. USE WITHIN 3-4 MONTHS.

RICH BLEND

- ADD THE CHOPPED KALE TO A BLENDER WITH THE WATER AND BLEND UNTIL SMOOTH.

- ADD THE HEMP SEEDS, BANANA, CACAO, AND VANILLA SEEDS, THEN BLEND AGAIN UNTIL SMOOTH AND CREAMY. SERVE IMMEDIATELY, WITH A PINCH OF RAW CACAO TO GARNISH.

ACAI

KNOCKOUT

THIS IS A GREAT ENERGY BOOSTER—PERFECT FOR BREAKFAST OR AN AFTERNOON PICK-ME-UP.

Ingredients

2 ¾ cups SPINACH

2 teaspoons açai powder

2 teaspoons MANUKA HONEY

PINCH GROUND CINNAMON

1 cup almond milk

crushed ice, to serve (optional)

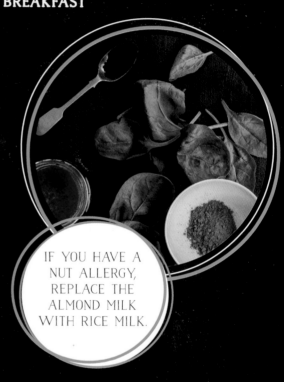

IF YOU HAVE A NUT ALLERGY, REPLACE THE ALMOND MILK WITH RICE MILK.

MAKE THIS SMOOTHIE

- PUT THE SPINACH, AÇAI POWDER, HONEY, AND CINNAMON INTO A BLENDER.

- POUR IN THE ALMOND MILK AND BLEND UNTIL SMOOTH AND CREAMY.

- STIR WELL, POUR OVER THE CRUSHED ICE, IF USING, AND SERVE IMMEDIATELY.

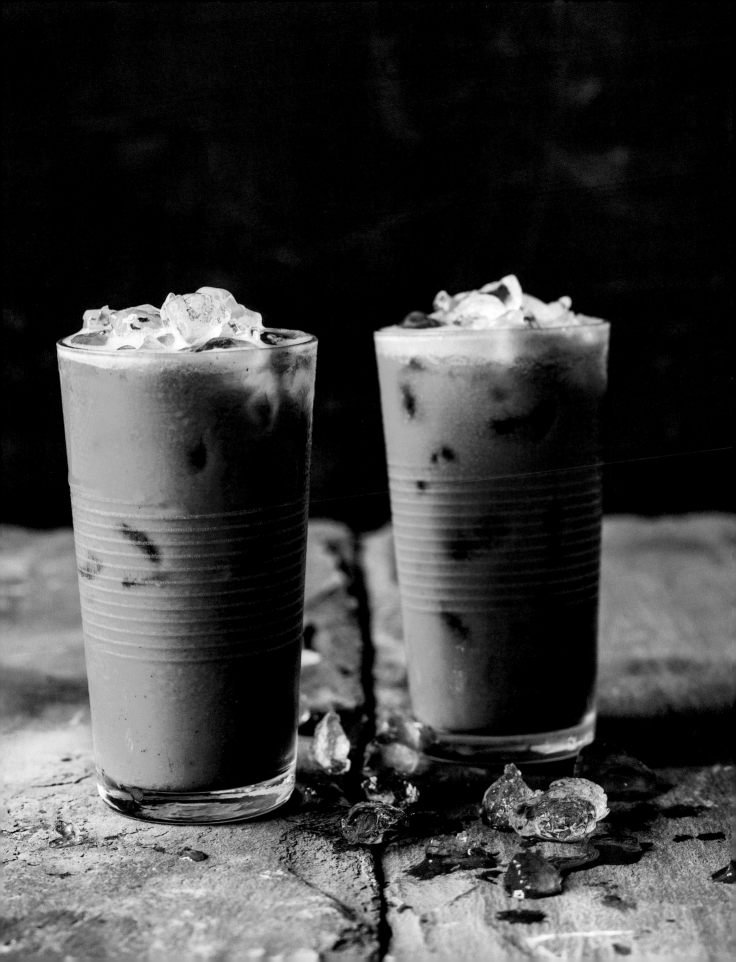

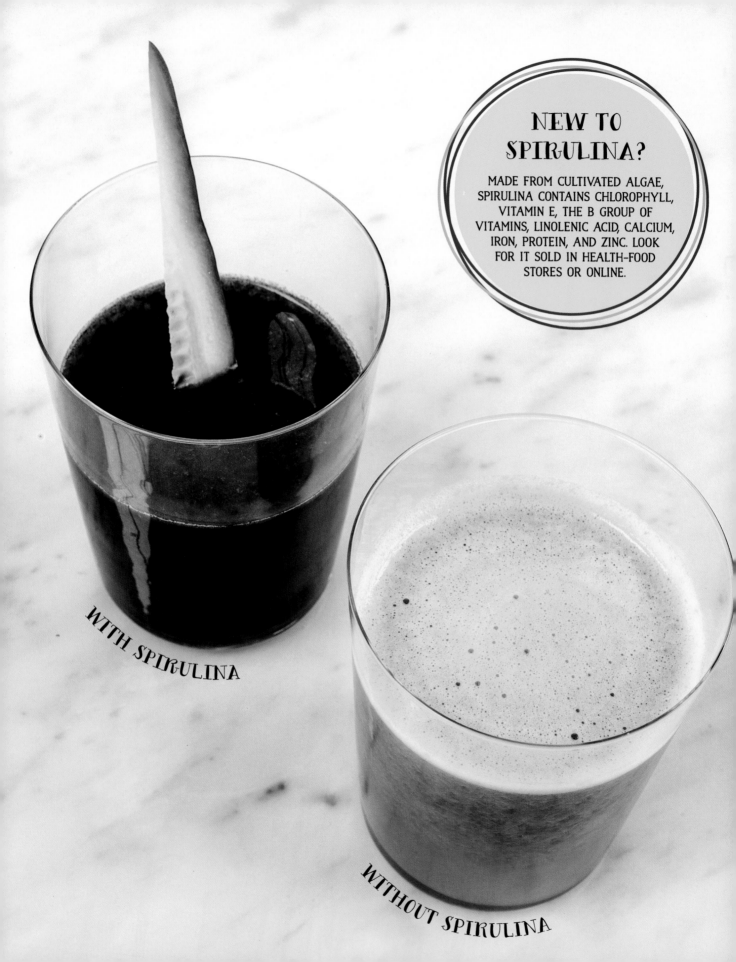

NEW TO SPIRULINA?

MADE FROM CULTIVATED ALGAE, SPIRULINA CONTAINS CHLOROPHYLL, VITAMIN E, THE B GROUP OF VITAMINS, LINOLENIC ACID, CALCIUM, IRON, PROTEIN, AND ZINC. LOOK FOR IT SOLD IN HEALTH-FOOD STORES OR ONLINE.

WITH SPIRULINA

WITHOUT SPIRULINA

GREEN STEAM

SERVES 1

BECAUSE MELON CONTAINS SUCH A HIGH PROPORTION OF WATER, IT IS GREAT FOR REHYDRATING. THE ADDITION OF SPIRULINA, WHICH CONTAINS BLOOD-CLEANSING CHLOROPHYLL, MAKES THIS JUICE PERFECT FOR PURIFYING THE SYSTEM.

Ingredients

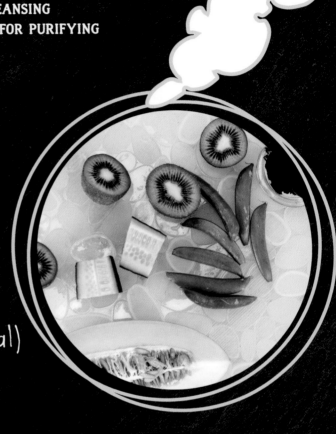

1⅓ cups SUGAR SNAP PEAS

2-inch PIECE OF CUCUMBER, PLUS A CUCUMBER STICK TO GARNISH

2 KIWIS, PEELED

¼ HONEYDEW MELON, PEELED AND THICKLY SLICED

1 teaspoon spirulina powder (optional)

1 cup chilled water

small handful ice (optional)

STIR IT UP

- FEED THE SUGAR SNAP PEAS, CUCUMBER, AND KIWIS INTO A JUICER, FOLLOWED BY THE MELON.

- STIR IN THE SPIRULINA POWDER, IF USING, AND FILL WITH THE WATER.

- FILL A GLASS HALFWAY WITH ICE, IF USING, THEN POUR IN THE JUICE AND SERVE IMMEDIATELY WITH A CUCUMBER STICK FOR A STIRRER.

SPRING CLEAN

THIS DARK JUICE TASTES SURPRISINGLY FRESH. WHEATGRASS HAS LONG BEEN RECOGNIZED FOR ITS DETOXIFYING AND HEALING PROPERTIES.

SERVES 1

Ingredients

1½ CUPS LARGE BROCCOLI, FLORETS

2 APPLES, HALVED

1 ZUCCHINI, HALVED

1 teaspoon wheatgrass powder

Small handful ice

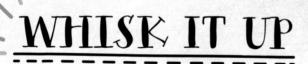

WONDERFUL WHEATGRASS

WHEATGRASS IS RICH IN CHLOROPHYLL AND PROTEIN, AND CONTAINS VITAMINS A, C, E, K, AND B12 PLUS A RANGE OF MINERALS. IT IS OFTEN SOLD IN HEALTH FOOD STORES AND JUICE BARS AS A QUICK AND CLEANSING 'SHOT'.

WHISK IT UP

- FEED THE BROCCOLI, APPLES, AND ZUCCHINI THROUGH A JUICER.

- ADD THE WHEATGRASS POWDER AND WHISK UNTIL SMOOTH.

- FILL A GLASS HALFWAY WITH ICE, POUR IN THE JUICE, AND SERVE IMMEDIATELY.

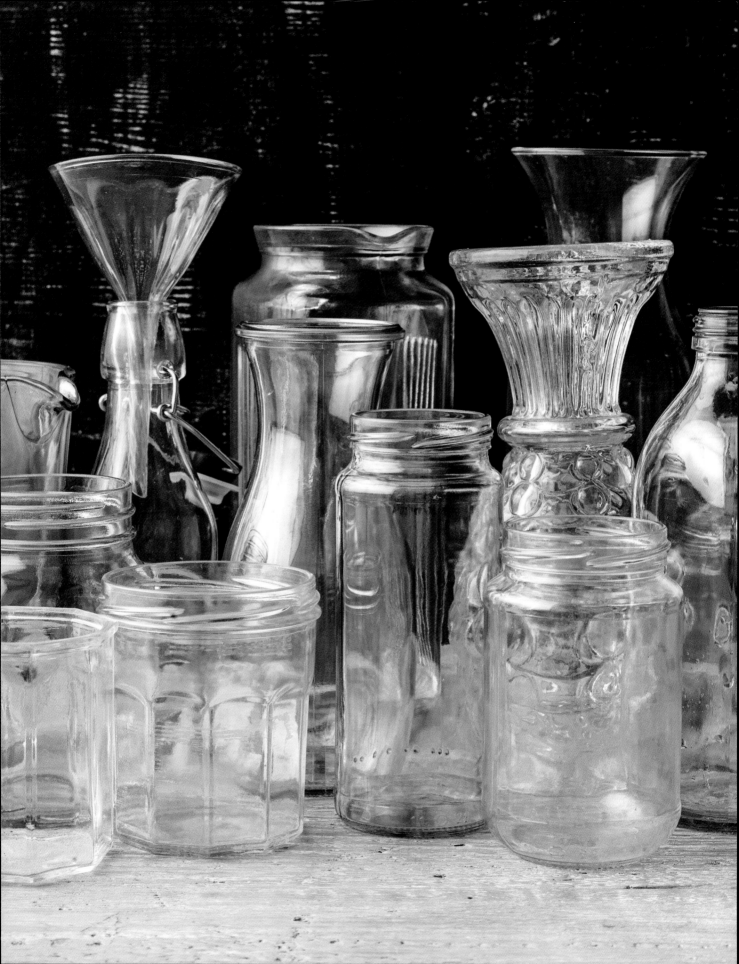

MANGO CLEANSER

SERVES 1

ADDING A BOOST POWDER TO YOUR SHOTS WILL ENSURE GOOD LEVELS OF NUTRIENT DENSITY, SO DON'T LEAVE THEM OUT.

Ingredients

$\frac{1}{2}$ CUP SPINACH

$\frac{1}{3}$ CUP PEELED MANGO CHUNKS

6 FRESH MINT LEAVES, PLUS EXTRA TO GARNISH

$\frac{1}{2}$ teaspoon BARLEYGRASS POWDER

$\frac{1}{2}$ cup chilled water

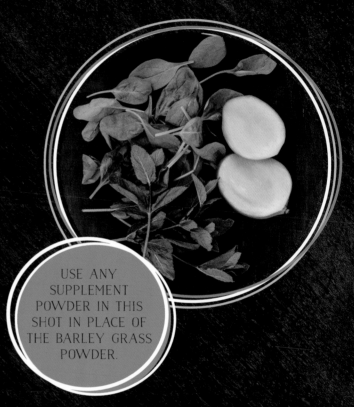

USE ANY SUPPLEMENT POWDER IN THIS SHOT IN PLACE OF THE BARLEY GRASS POWDER.

BLEND!

- PUT THE SPINACH, MANGO, MINT, AND BARLEY GRASS POWDER INTO A BLENDER.

- POUR IN THE WATER AND BLEND UNTIL SMOOTH. SERVE IMMEDIATELY, GARNISHED WITH MINT LEAVES.

CUCUMBER & APPLE CHARGER

REFRESHING AND ZINGY, CUCUMBER AND APPLE MAKE A GREAT DUO IN THIS RECHARGING SHOT.

SERVES 1

CELERY IS A GREAT SUBSTITUTE FOR CUCUMBER— JUST ADD A LITTLE EXTRA WATER WHEN BLENDING.

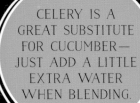
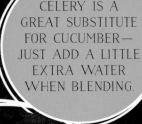

Ingredients

¹⁄₆ SMAL GREEN APPLE

¹⁄₈ CUCUMBER

juice ½ lime, plus a small wedge to garnish

½ teaspoon chlorophyll powder

3 ½ tablespoons chilled water

BLEND!

- PEEL AND COARSELY CHOP THE APPLE AND COARSELY CHOP THE CUCUMBER, THEN PUT INTO A BLENDER WITH THE LIME JUICE AND CHLOROPHYLL POWDER.

- POUR IN THE WATER AND BLEND UNTIL SMOOTH. SERVE IMMEDIATELY WITH A SMALL WEDGE OF LIME.

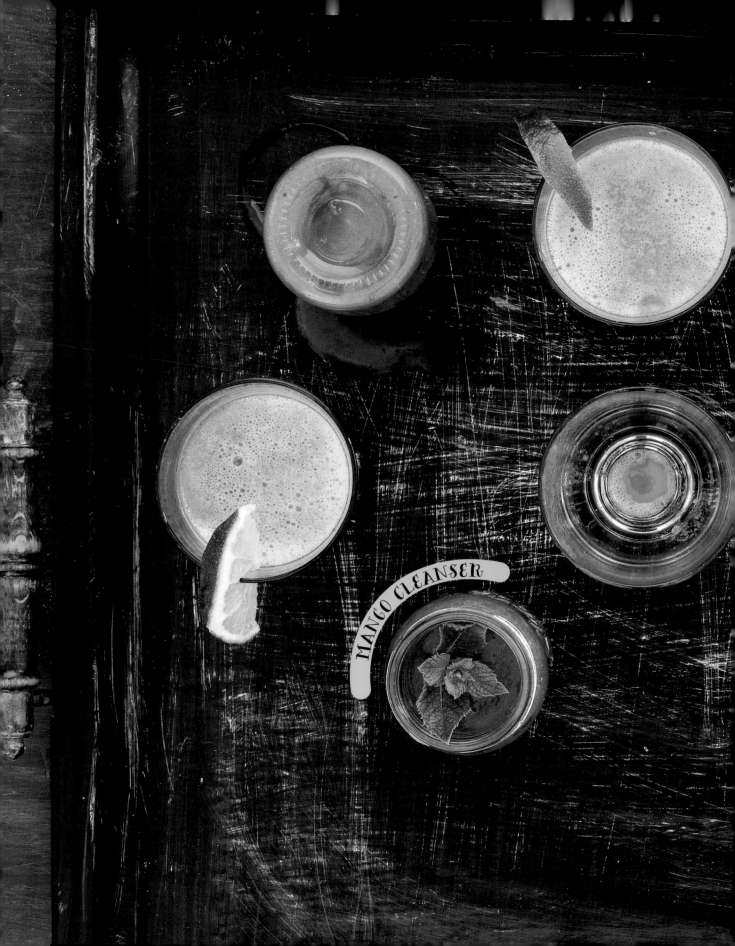

MANGO CLEANSER

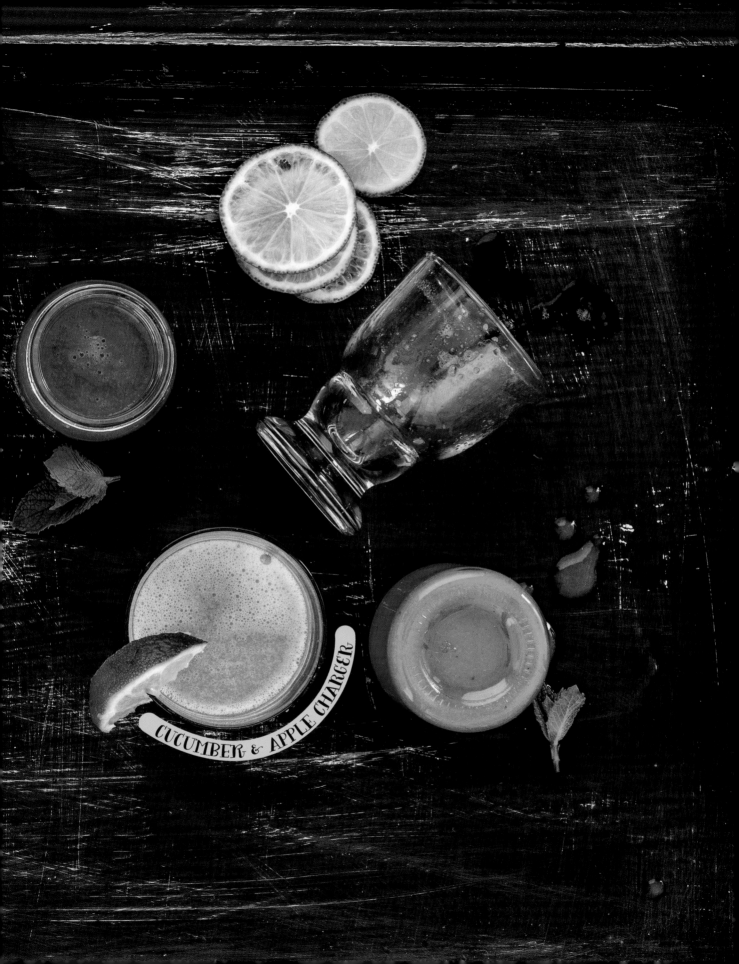

CUCUMBER & APPLE CHARGER

DANDELION SUNRISE

SERVES 1

COCONUT BUTTER IS A SPREAD MADE FROM THE FLESH OF THE COCONUT IN THE SAME WAY THAT PEANUTS ARE USED TO MAKE PEANUT BUTTER. IT'S PACKED WITH HEALTHY FATS AND HELPS TO KEEP YOU FULLER FOR LONGER WHEN ADDED TO SMOOTHIES.

Ingredients

½ cup DANDELION GREENS

¾ cup CURLY GREEN KALE

1 cup chilled water

½ cup CASHEW NUTS

1 ½ teaspoons COCONUT BUTTER

1 tablespoon SUNFLOWER SEEDS

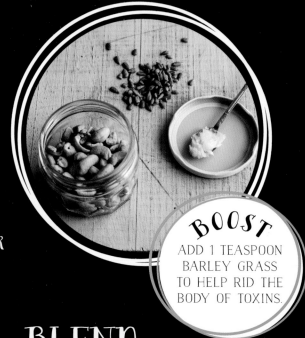

BOOST
ADD 1 TEASPOON BARLEY GRASS TO HELP RID THE BODY OF TOXINS.

READY STEADY...BLEND

- PUT THE DANDELION GREENS, KALE, AND WATER INTO A BLENDER AND BLEND UNTIL SMOOTH.

- ADD THE CASHEW NUTS, COCONUT BUTTER, AND SUNFLOWER SEEDS, AND BLEND UNTIL SMOOTH AND CREAMY. SERVE IMMEDIATELY.

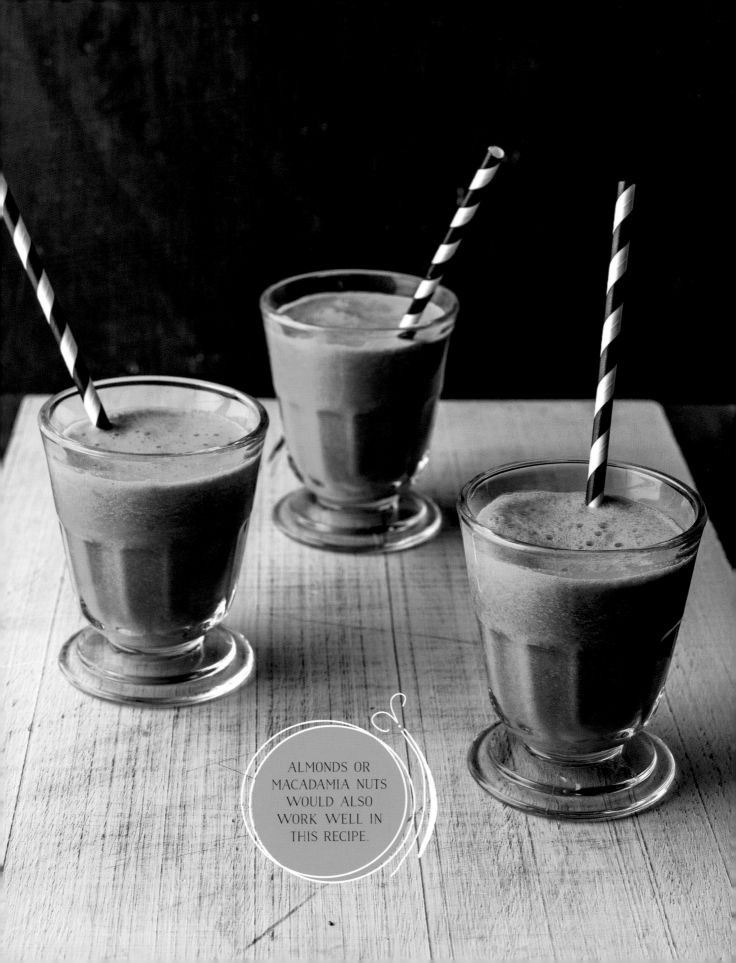

ALMONDS OR
MACADAMIA NUTS
WOULD ALSO
WORK WELL IN
THIS RECIPE.

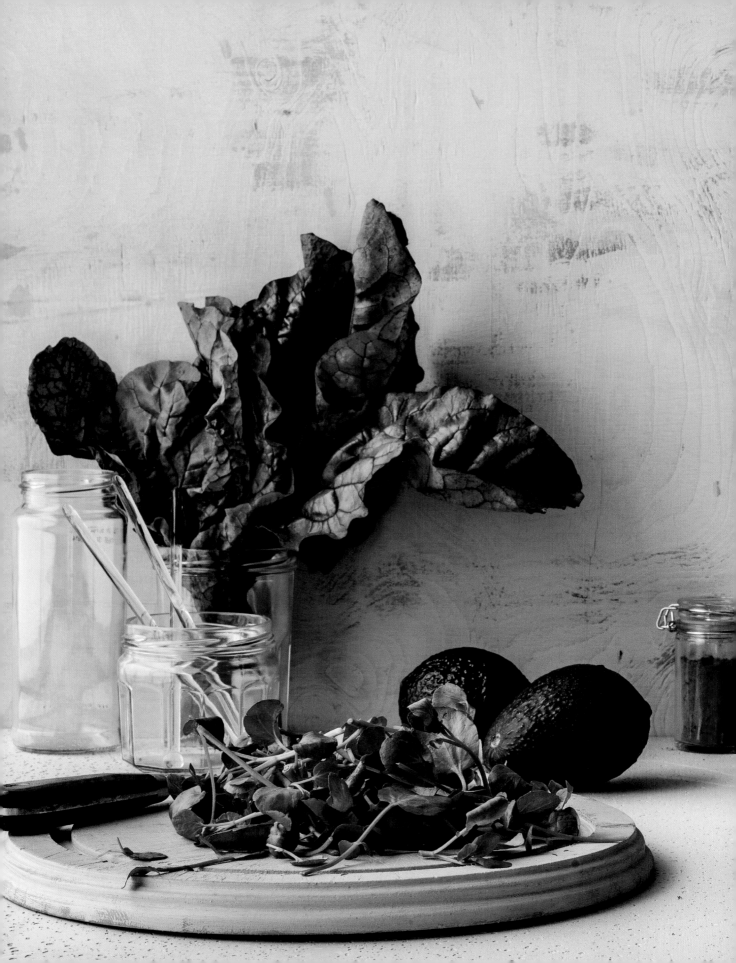

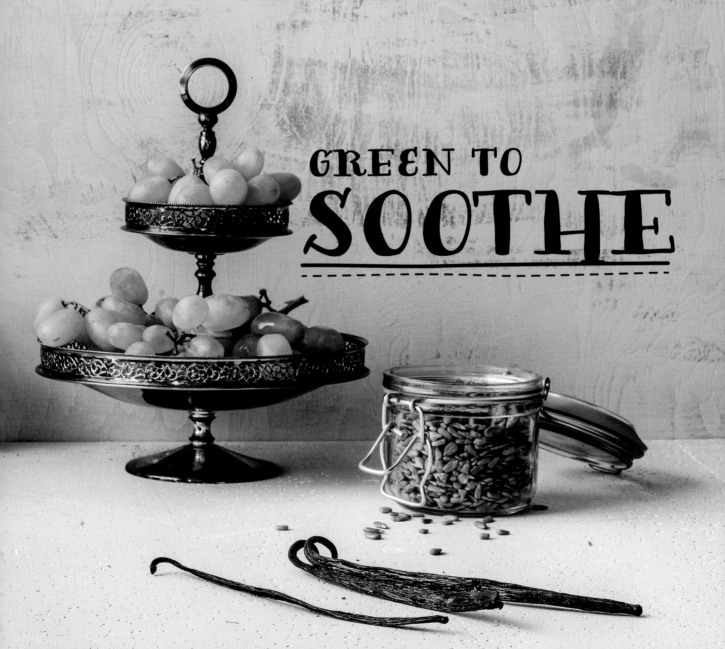

GREEN TO
SOOTHE

SUPERSMOOTHIE

THE AVOCADO IS A NUTRIENT-DENSE FOOD THAT HELPS THE BODY TO ABSORB FAT-SOLUBLE NUTRIENTS. IF THAT ISN'T ENOUGH TO PERSUADE YOU TO ADD AVOCADOS TO SMOOTHIES, DO IT BECAUSE IT MAKES THEM CREAMY AND SOOTHING!

Ingredients

1 cup SPINACH

1 cup cooled licorice tea

½ AVOCADO, PITTED AND FLESH SCOOPED FROM SKIN

1 FROZEN BANANA

1 teaspoon chia seeds, plus extra to garnish

WHEN YOU HAVE AN ABUNDANCE OF FRUIT AND VEGETABLES, FREEZE THEM IN SMALL PORTIONS AND THEY'RE READY TO GO FOR YOUR SMOOTHIES.

MIX!

- BLEND THE SPINACH AND LICORICE TEA IN A BLENDER UNTIL SMOOTH.

- CHOP THE AVOCADO, ADD IT TO THE BLENDER WITH THE BANANA AND CHIA SEEDS, AND BLEND UNTIL SMOOTH AND CREAMY. SERVE IMMEDIATELY, GARNISHED WITH A SPRINKLE OF CHIA SEEDS.

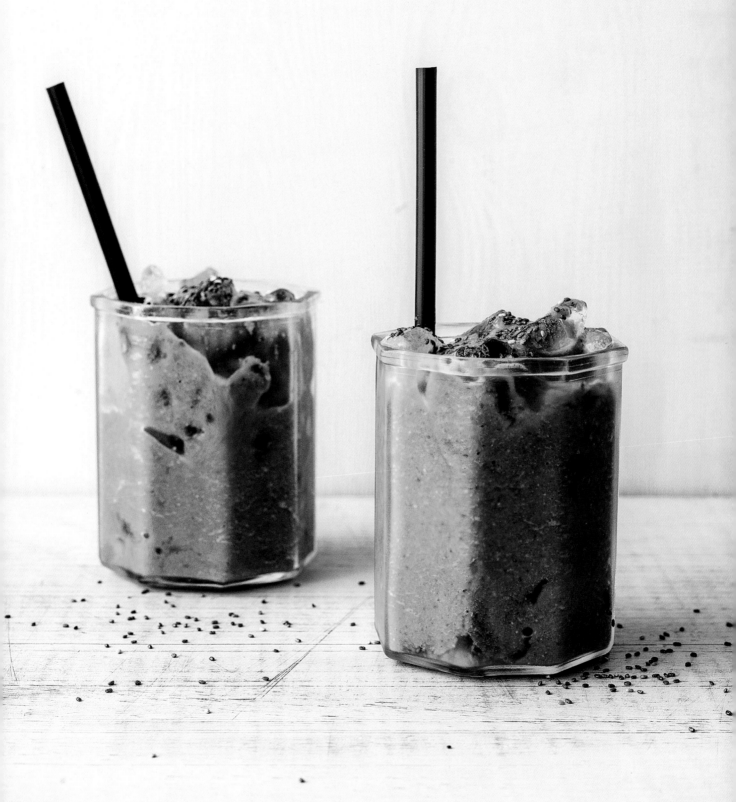

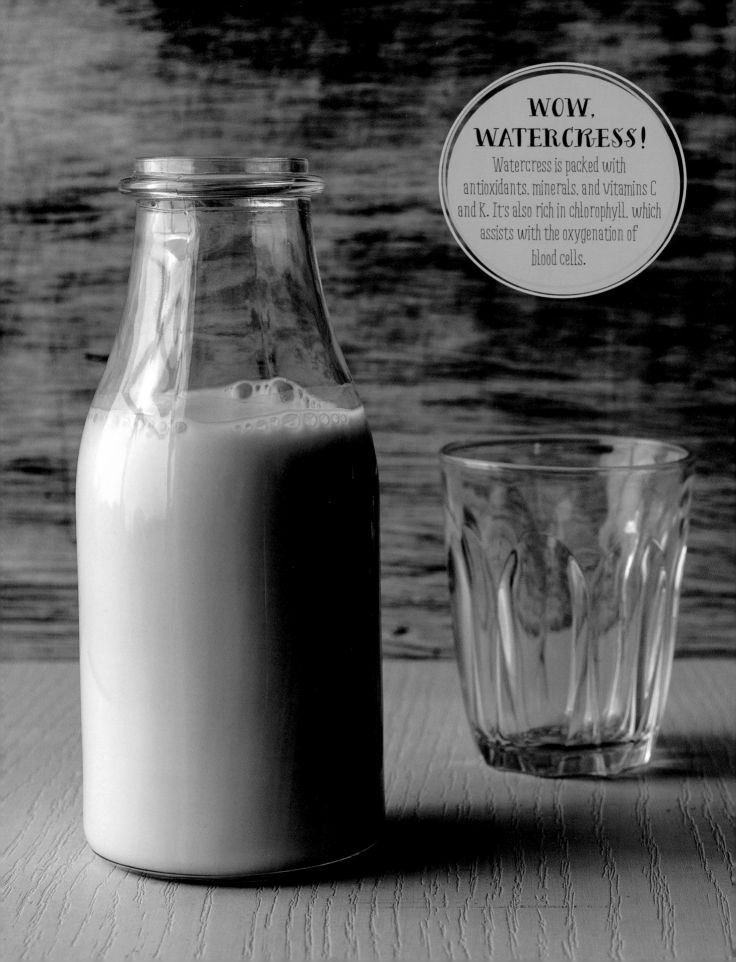

WOW, WATERCRESS!

Watercress is packed with antioxidants, minerals, and vitamins C and K. It's also rich in chlorophyll, which assists with the oxygenation of blood cells.

TURBO RECHARGER

SERVES 1   THIS SMOOTHIE INCLUDES EVERYTHING YOU NEED TO REVITALIZE YOUR BODY: REHYDRATING MELON, ENERGY-BOOSTING BANANA, VITAMIN C-PACKED GRAPES, AND IRON-RICH WATERCRESS.

Ingredients

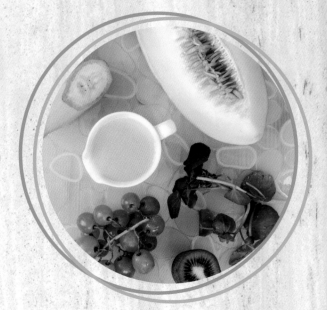

½ HONEYDEW MELON, PEELED, SEEDED, AND COARSELY CHOPPED

1 BANANA, PEELED AND COARSELY CHOPPED

1 KIWI, PEELED AND COARSELY CHOPPED

¾ CUP GREEN SEEDLESS GRAPES

SMALL HANDFUL WATERCRESS

½ CUP unsweetened rice, almond, or soy milk

small handful crushed ice (optional)

POWER UP

- PUT THE MELON, BANANA, KIWI, GRAPES, AND WATERCRESS INTO A BLENDER AND BLEND.

- ADD THE MILK AND CRUSHED ICE, IF USING, AND BLEND AGAIN, UNTIL SMOOTH.

- POUR INTO A GLASS AND SERVE IMMEDIATELY.

CUCUMBER SOOTHER

SERVES 1

THIS FRESH AND LIGHT JUICE WITH ITS ALOE VERA ADDITION CAN HELP TO REDUCE PROBLEMS SUCH AS HEARTBURN.

Ingredients

1 LARGE PEAR

⅓ CUCUMBER, PLUS A SLICE TO GARNISH

1 GREEN APPLE

¼ CUP FRESH MINT, PLUS A SPRIG TO GARNISH

1 tablespoon aloe vera gel

crushed ice, to serve (optional)

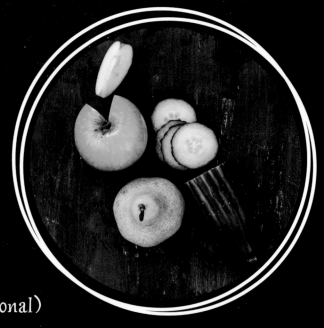

TO MAKE THIS JUICE

- COARSELY CHOP THE PEAR, CUCUMBER, AND APPLE, THEN FEED INTO THE FUNNEL OF A JUICER WITH THE MINT AND JUICE.

- STIR IN THE ALOE VERA GEL UNTIL COMBINED. POUR THE CRUSHED ICE, IF USING, INTO A GLASS, THEN POUR IN THE JUICE. SERVE IMMEDIATELY, GARNISHED WITH A CUCUMBER SLICE AND A SPRIG OF MINT.

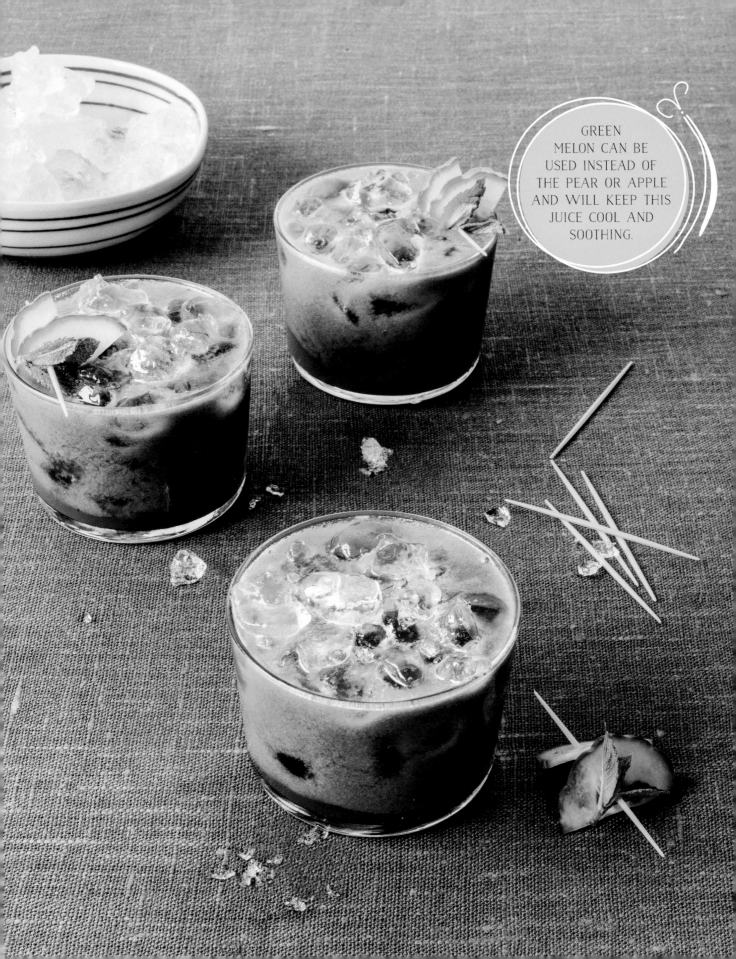

GREEN MELON CAN BE USED INSTEAD OF THE PEAR OR APPLE AND WILL KEEP THIS JUICE COOL AND SOOTHING.

GREEK GREEN

SERVES 1

Ingredients

¼ CUP SHREDDED CURLY GREEN KALE

1 cup chilled water

¼ VANILLA BEAN, SEEDS SCRAPED

½ CUP GREEK-STYLE YOGURT

⅓ CUP COCONUT FLESH

1 tablespoon ALMOND BUTTER

MAKE IT SMOOTH!

- ADD THE SHREDDED KALE TO A BLENDER WITH THE WATER AND BLEND UNTIL SMOOTH AND CREAMY.

- ADD THE VANILLA SEEDS TO THE BLENDER WITH THE YOGURT, COCONUT, AND ALMOND BUTTER AND BLEND UNTIL SMOOTH. SERVE IMMEDIATELY.

MELLOW MR. GREEN

SERVES 1

Ingredients

½ CUP ARUGULA

1 cup chilled water

1 KIWI, PEELED

1 CUP PEELED AND SEEDED CANTELOUPE CHUNKS

3 tablespoons COCONUT CREAM

2 teaspoons PEANUT BUTTER

BLEND IT!

- PUT THE ARUGULA AND WATER INTO A BLENDER AND BLEND UNTIL SMOOTH.

- CHOP THE KIWI AND MELON, THEN ADD TO THE BLENDER WITH THE COCONUT CREAM AND PEANUT BUTTER. BLEND UNTIL CREAMY. SERVE IMMEDIATELY.

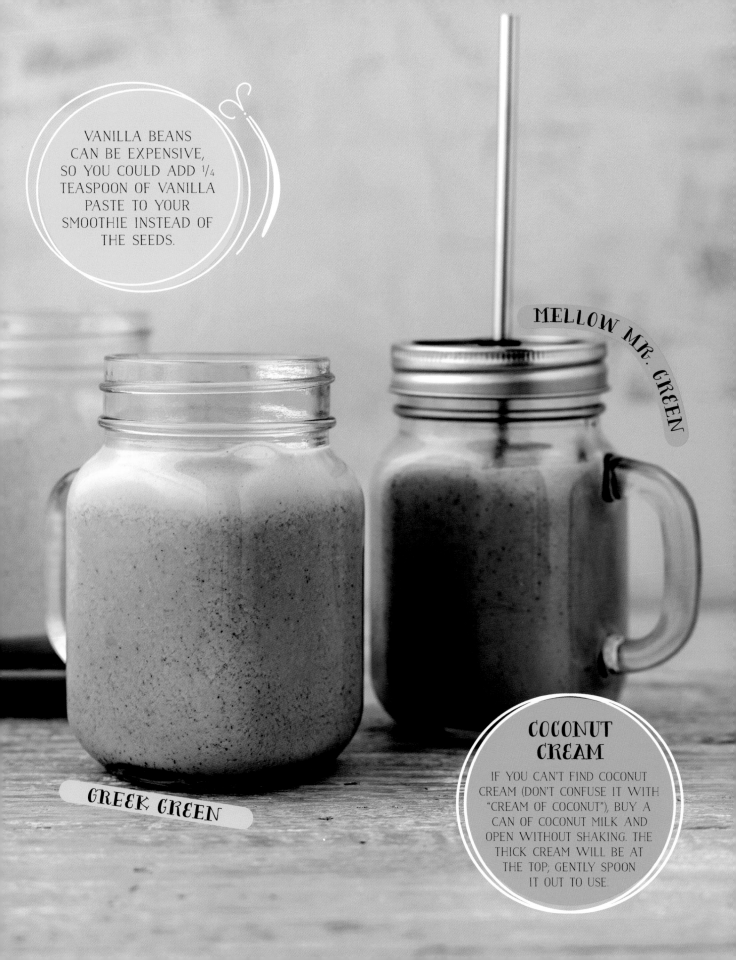

VANILLA BEANS
CAN BE EXPENSIVE,
SO YOU COULD ADD ¼
TEASPOON OF VANILLA
PASTE TO YOUR
SMOOTHIE INSTEAD OF
THE SEEDS.

MELLOW MR. GREEN

GREEK GREEN

COCONUT CREAM

IF YOU CAN'T FIND COCONUT
CREAM (DON'T CONFUSE IT WITH
"CREAM OF COCONUT"), BUY A
CAN OF COCONUT MILK AND
OPEN WITHOUT SHAKING. THE
THICK CREAM WILL BE AT
THE TOP; GENTLY SPOON
IT OUT TO USE.

PINEAPPLE PUMP

PERFECT FOR WHEN YOU WANT SOMETHING TO QUENCH YOUR THIRST WITH A FRUITY TWIST. THE PINEAPPLE AND MINT IN THIS RECIPE ARE A WINNING COMBINATION.

FOR ANOTHER FRUITY OPTION, TRY PAPAYA IN PLACE OF THE PINEAPPLE.

— Ingredients

5 CELERY STALKS

2 CUPS CHOPPED CURLY GREEN KALE PLUS EXTRA TO GARNISH

1 CUP PEELED AND CORED FRESH PINEAPPLE CHUNKS, PLUS EXTRA TO GARNISH

2/3 CUP MINT

1 teaspoon wheatgrass powder

BOOST

ADD A SMALL PIECE OF TURMERIC ROOT TO HELP RELIEVE INFLAMED JOINTS.

MIX IT UP

- COARSELY CHOP THE CELERY, FEED INTO THE JUICER FUNNEL WITH THE KALE, PINEAPPLE, MINT, AND JUICE.

- STIR IN THE WHEATGRASS POWDER UNTIL COMBINED. SERVE IMMEDIATELY, GARNISHED WITH A SMALL WEDGE OF PINEAPPLE AND A LEAF OF KALE.

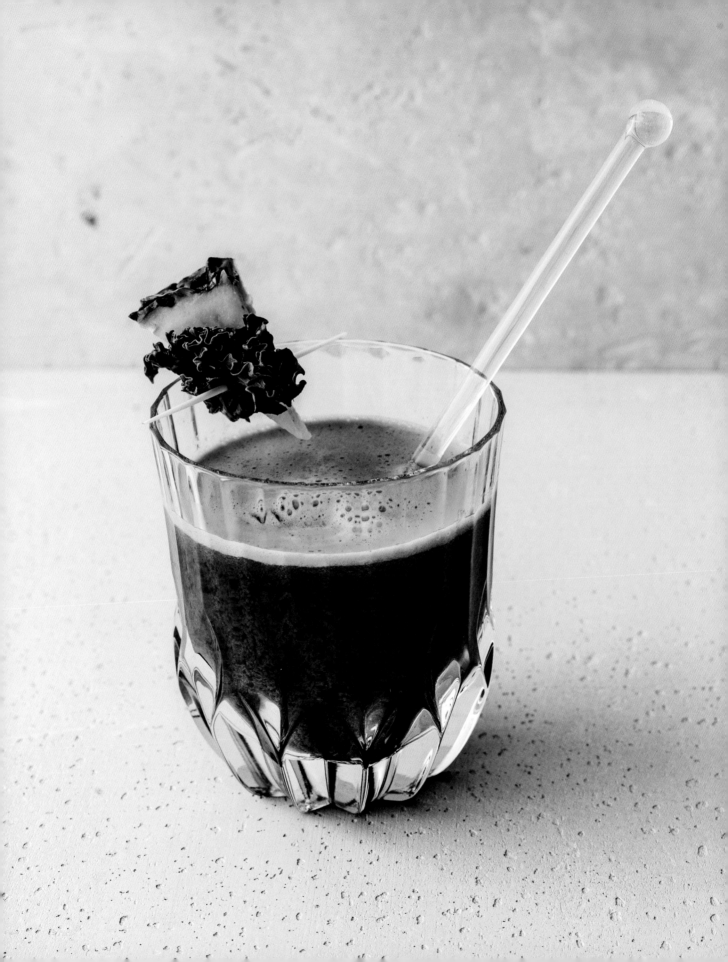

THE SPECIAL INGREDIENTS

THAT WILL HELP KEEP YOUR DIGESTIVE SYSTEM HEALTHY

Indulging in a beautiful smoothie when you've got digestive problems works in two ways—it can help comfort, relax, and soothe you as you drink, and it can have a range of real health benefits for your digestive tract. Here's how.

HELP EASE INDIGESTION/HEARTBURN/DYSPEPSIA/ULCERS

* Smoothies are an ideal way to eat if you experience indigestion or heartburn, because the blending process breaks down the foods into tiny particles that are easier to digest, while retaining all the nutrients and fiber.
* Smoothies are high in fiber, and some studies show that a high-fiber diet is associated with a lower risk of acid reflux (GERD)—although citrus fruit and spices can irritate the condition so the advice is to avoid these.
* Manuka honey helps prevent or eliminate *Helicobacter pylori*, bacteria found in the stomach that can cause dyspepsia, stomach ulcers, and stomach cancer. The honey can also help relieve acid reflux, indigestion. and gastritis.
* Licorice root has long been used in folk medicine to soothe the digestive system and as a treatment for peptic and stomach ulcers.

HELP ABSORB NUTRIENTS IN THE DIGESTIVE TRACT

By blending or juicing (particularly with the new-style, high-speed personal blenders) you are making it easier for your body to absorb the nutrients in the ingredients. Pulverizing the fibrous tissues and cells maximizes the amount of nutrients your body receives and uses.

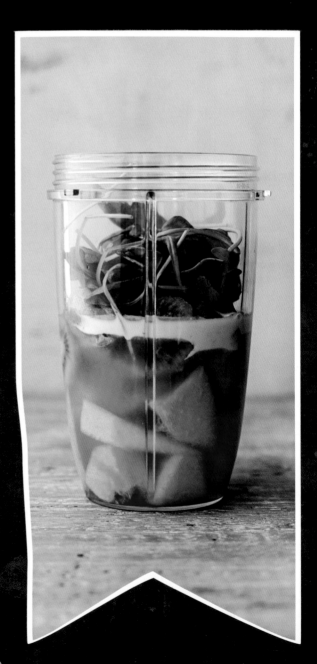

HELP PREVENT IRRITABLE BOWEL SYNDROME (IBS)

Boost your internal bacteria. Probiotics are often called "friendly bacteria"—they occur naturally in the digestive tract and can ease bloating and gas. Adding live yogurt, which contains millions of these bacteria, to your drinks should help boost your levels

Prebiotics are types of indigestible carbohydrate that probiotics feed on, so levels of friendly bacteria may be increased by eating foods that contain them. Prebiotic-rich foods include bananas, asparagus, and artichokes

Some people find that cereals and grains cause bloating and irritable bowel syndrome. If that's the case, get your fiber from fruit and vegetables instead

It's important to keep drinking, especially water. It encourages the passage of waste through your digestive system and helps soften stools, so drinking smoothies and juices is an ideal way to keep flushing through your system

Try aloe vera, which has long been used in herbal medicine to calm the digestive tract and is ideal for helping irritable bowel syndrome and digestive disorders

Mint is known to calm the digestive tract, relieving indigestion, and has also been linked with improvement in irritable bowel syndrome symptoms, while pectin-rich apples have been shown to help control a loose bowel.

BEAT CONSTIPATION

If you experience constipation, you need a high-fiber, high-fluids diet. A mix of both smoothies and juices may be ideal because smoothies keep all the fiber in the produce, while juices have a higher liquid content. Some of the highest-fiber foods for your smoothies are peas, mangoes, papaya, apricots, figs, berries, coconut flesh, avocados, broccoli, carrots, fennel, kale, spinach, and watercress.

Fruits with a particularly high water content include watermelon (at 92 percent), canteloupe, strawberries, grapefruit, peaches, pineapple, oranges, and raspberries. And high-water vegetables include cucumber and lettuce (at 96 percent), zucchini, radishes, celery, tomatoes, and cabbage.

Olive oil, chiles, ginger, and licorice have all been used for centuries to help keep you regular by speeding up the passage of food through the digestive system.

CREAMY AVOCADOS TO IMPROVE DIGESTION HEALTH

Using avocados to give your smoothies a gorgeous nondairy creamy texture is a great idea for your digestive health. One avocado contains around 1 ounce of healthy fats, over half of which is oleic acid. This fat not only helps the pancreas produce digestive enzymes, but also helps the digestive tract increase absorption of carotenes, which convert to vitamin A in the body—a vitamin that both repairs and maintains the delicate lining of the intestines.

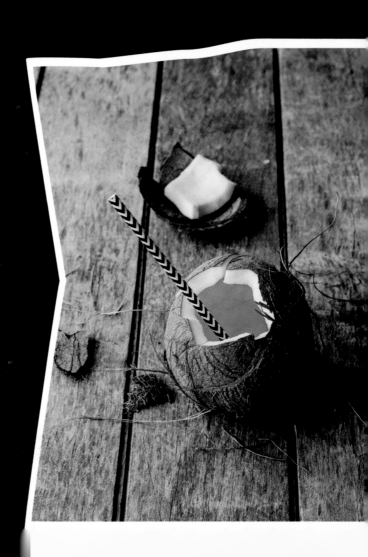

GO NUTS!

SMOOTH AND CREAMY MEETS SWEET AND NUTTY IN THIS DELICIOUS PICK-ME-UP.

SERVES 1

Ingredients

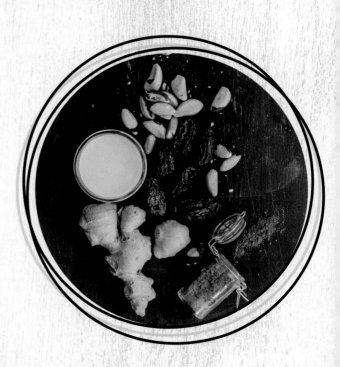

½ AVOCADO, PITTED AND FLESH SCOOPED FROM SKIN

4 BRAZIL NUTS

3 MEDJOOL DATES

¼-inch FRESH GINGER, PEELED

1 ½ cups almond milk

¼ teaspoon cinnamon, plus a pinch to garnish

crushed ice, to serve (optional)

BLEND IT!

- PUT THE AVOCADO, NUTS, DATES, AND GINGER INTO A BLENDER.

- POUR IN THE ALMOND MILK, ADD THE CINNAMON, AND BLEND AGAIN UNTIL SMOOTH.

- POUR OVER CRUSHED ICE, IF USING, AND SERVE IMMEDIATELY, SPRINKLED WITH A LITTLE CINNAMON.

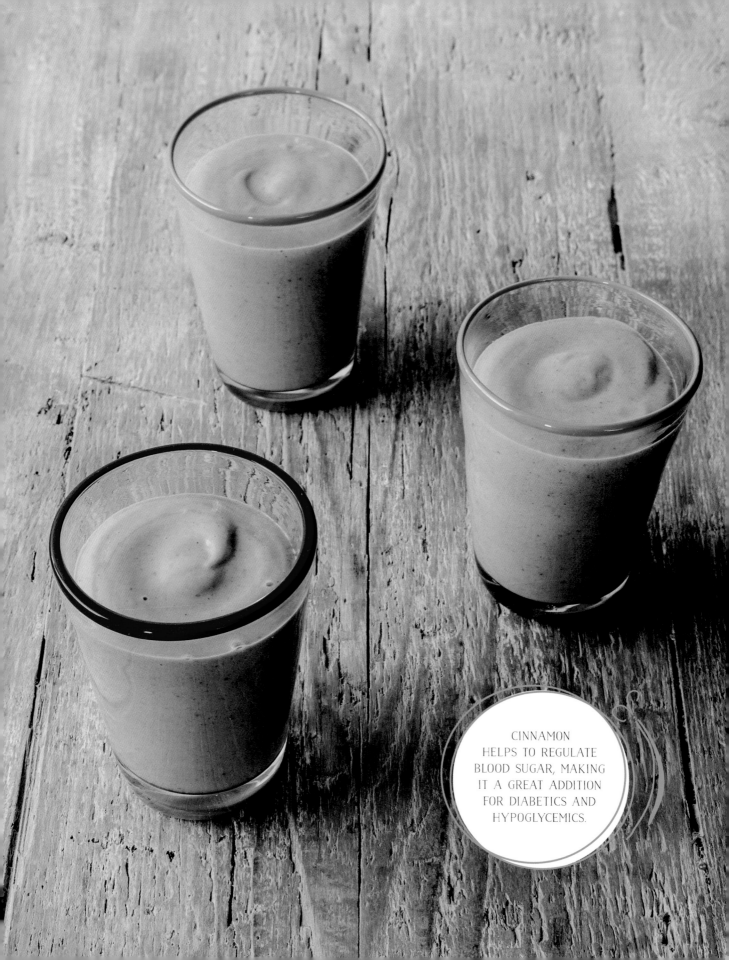

CINNAMON
HELPS TO REGULATE
BLOOD SUGAR, MAKING
IT A GREAT ADDITION
FOR DIABETICS AND
HYPOGLYCEMICS.

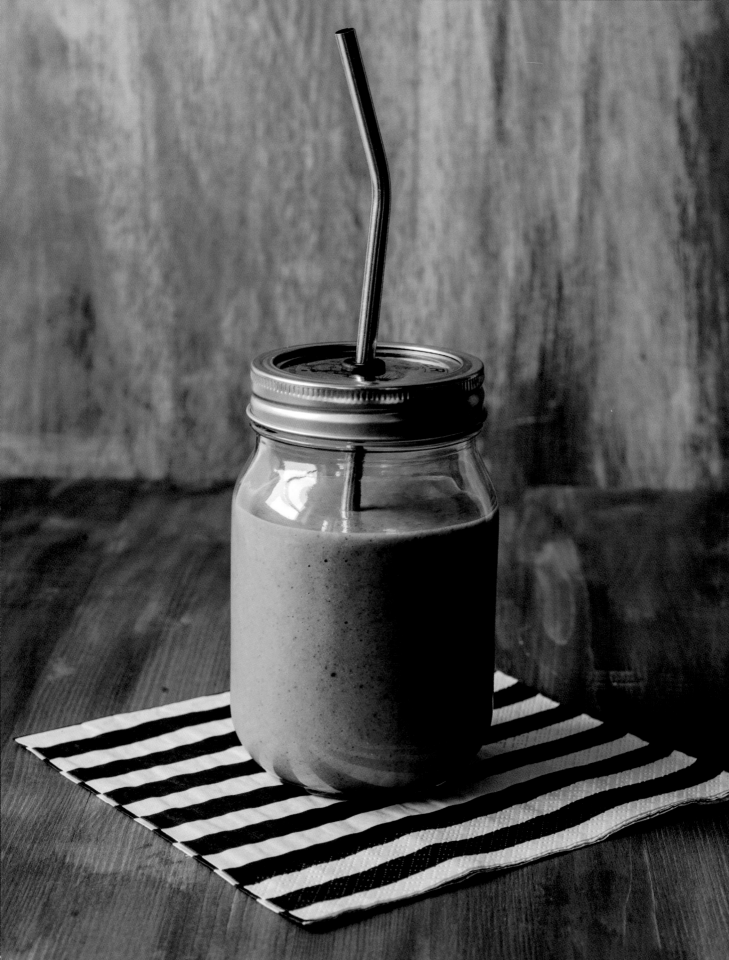

BROCCOLI BOOSTER

SERVES 1

BANANAS SUPPRESS ACID IN THE DIGESTIVE TRACT, WHICH ALLEVIATES HEARTBURN AND HELPS FIGHT ULCERS. THEY ALSO CONTAIN A SOLUBLE FIBER THAT AIDS THE ELIMINATION PROCESS, SO THEY ARE GREAT FOR BOOSTING DIGESTIVE HEALTH.

Ingredients

1 1/2 CUPS BROCCOLI STEM

2 3/4 CUPS SPINACH

1 CUP chilled water

1 FROZEN BANANA

1 tablespoon PUMPKIN SEED BUTTER

1 tablespoon MANUKA HONEY

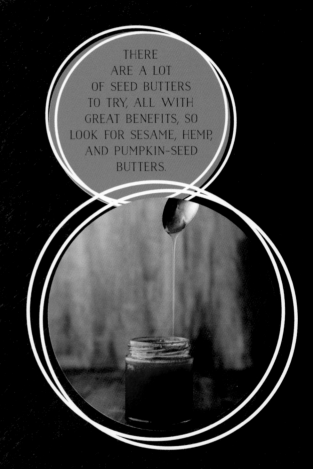

THERE ARE A LOT OF SEED BUTTERS TO TRY, ALL WITH GREAT BENEFITS, SO LOOK FOR SESAME, HEMP, AND PUMPKIN-SEED BUTTERS.

MIX IT UP

- BLEND THE BROCCOLI STEM WITH THE SPINACH AND WATER IN A BLENDER UNTIL SMOOTH.

- ADD THE BANANA, PUMPKIN-SEED BUTTER, AND HONEY, THEN BLEND AGAIN UNTIL SMOOTH AND CREAMY. SERVE IMMEDIATELY.

GREEN ENERGY

THIS SUPERSMOOTHIE IS PACKED WITH ANTIOXIDANTS, VITAMINS, AND MINERALS.

SERVES 1

Ingredients

1 PEAR, HALVED

1½ CUPS YOUNG SPINACH

4 SPRIGS FRESH FLAT-LEAF PARSLEY

¼ CUCUMBER, COARSELY CHOPPED

½ AVOCADO, PITTED AND FLESH SCOOPED FROM SKIN

½ teaspoon spirulina powder

chilled water, to taste

1 BRAZIL NUT, COARSELY CHOPPED

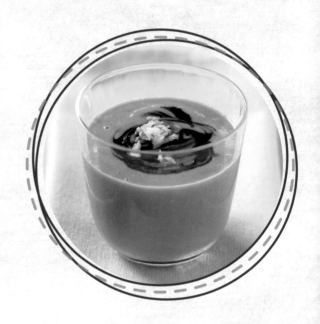

SWIRL IT!

- FEED THE PEAR THROUGH A JUICER.

- POUR THE PEAR JUICE INTO A BLENDER AND ADD THE SPINACH, PARSLEY, CUCUMBER, AND AVOCADO. BLEND AGAIN UNTIL SMOOTH.

- POUR INTO A GLASS. MIX THE SPIRULINA WITH JUST ENOUGH WATER TO MAKE A THICK LIQUID, THEN SWIRL THIS INTO THE JUICE.

- SPRINKLE WITH THE CHOPPED BRAZIL NUT, THEN SERVE.

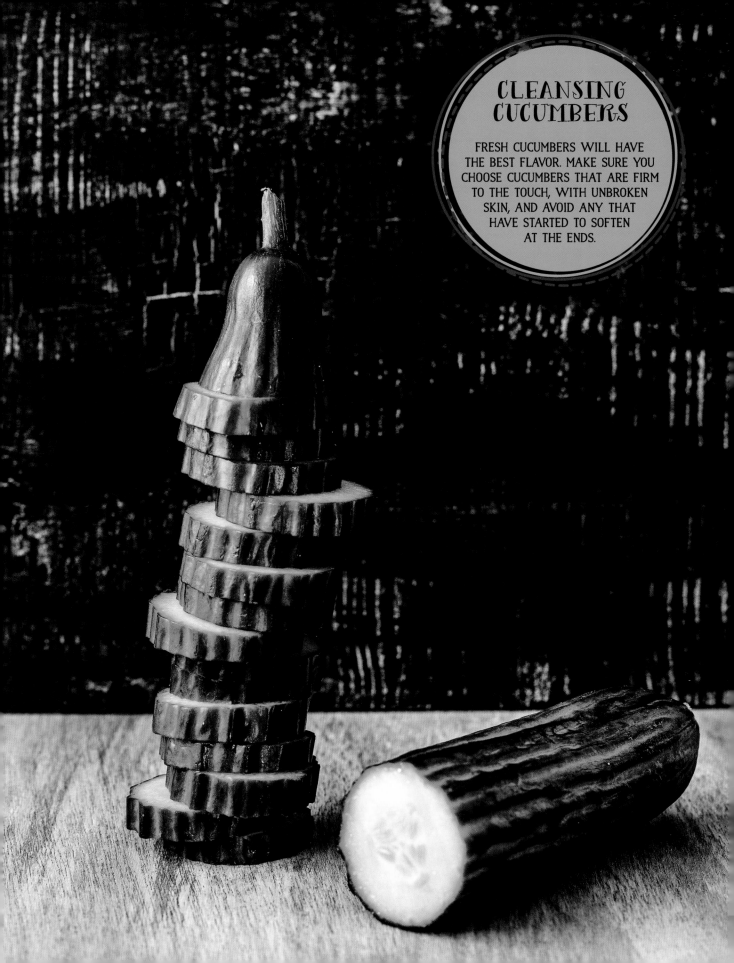

MINTED MELON JUICE

QUENCH YOUR THIRST WITH THE LIGHTEST OF FRUIT JUICES. FORGET SUGAR-LOADED COMMERCIAL SOFT DRINKS; THIS SIMPLE HOMEMADE ONE HAS JUST FOUR INGREDIENTS PLUS ICE AND IS ADDITIVE-FREE.

Ingredients

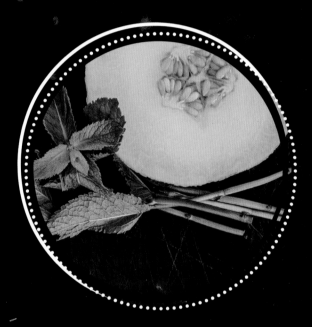

½ HONEYDEW MELON, PEELED AND THICKLY SLICED

5 STEMS FRESH MINT

½ LIME ZEST AND A LITTLE PITH REMOVED

1-inch SLICE BROCCOLI STEM

small handful crushed ice (optional)

JUICE IT

- FEED THE MELON, MINT, LIME, AND BROCCOLI THROUGH A JUICER.

- FILL A GLASS HALFWAY WITH CRUSHED ICE, IF USING, THEN POUR IN THE JUICE AND SERVE IMMEDIATELY.

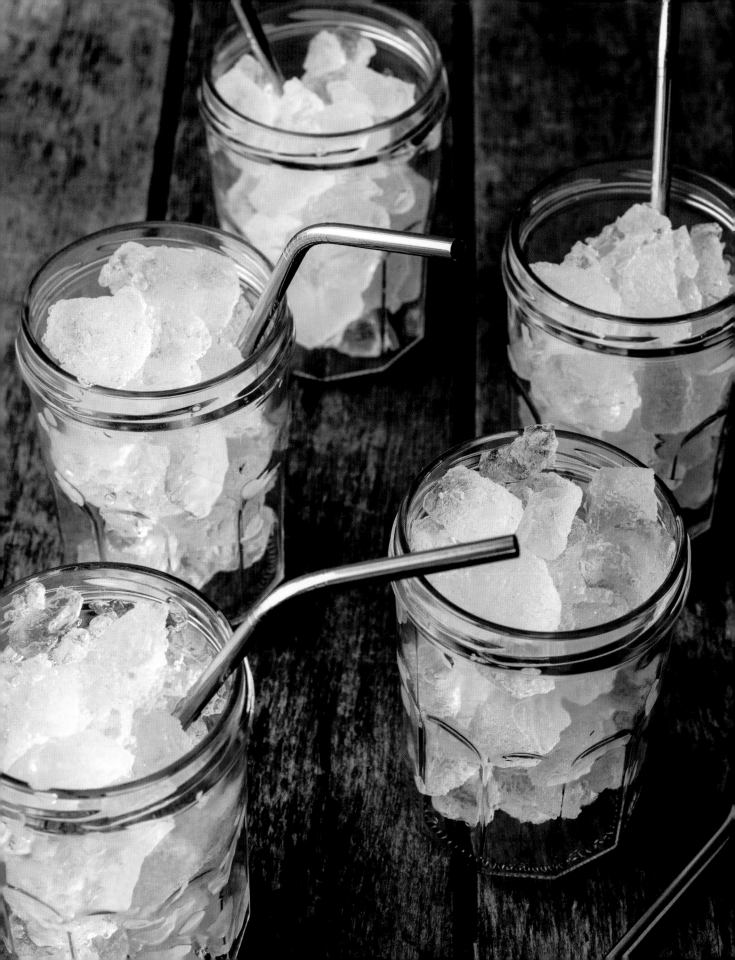

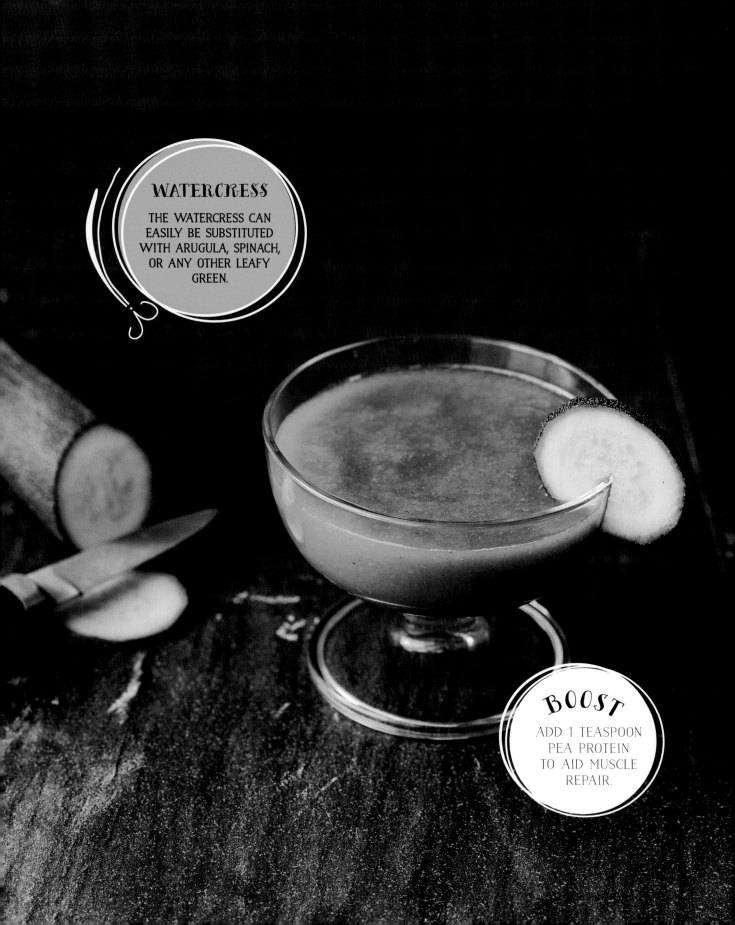

WATERCRESS

THE WATERCRESS CAN EASILY BE SUBSTITUTED WITH ARUGULA, SPINACH, OR ANY OTHER LEAFY GREEN.

BOOST

ADD 1 TEASPOON PEA PROTEIN TO AID MUSCLE REPAIR.

THE GRASSHOPPER

YOU'LL PROBABLY ALREADY HAVE MOST OF THE
INGREDIENTS FOR THIS SHOT IN YOUR REFRIGERATOR,
SO IT CAN BE WHIPPED UP IN AN INSTANT!

SERVES 1

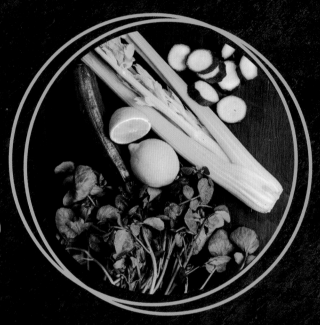

Ingredients

¼ CUP CHOPPED ZUCCHINI, PLUS
A SMALL SLICE TO GARNISH

1 SMALL CELERY STALK, CHOPPED

4 SPRIGS OF WATERCRESS

juice of ½ lemon

1 tablespoon chilled water

>TAKE A SHOT!<

- PUT THE CHOPPED ZUCCHINI AND CELERY INTO THE BLENDER.
  ADD THE WATERCRESS AND LEMON JUICE.

- POUR IN THE WATER AND BLEND UNTIL SMOOTH.
  SERVE IMMEDIATELY, GARNISHED WITH A SMALL
  SLICE OF ZUCCHINI.

SPINACH AID

DARK AND DREAMY, THIS SHOT PACKS A SUPERCHARGE
OF GOODNESS—DON'T LEAVE A SINGLE DROP!

SERVES 1

Ingredients

¾ CUP SPINACH

1 tablespoon aloe vera gel

juice of ½ lime

½ teaspoon spirulina powder

3 ½ tablespoons chilled water

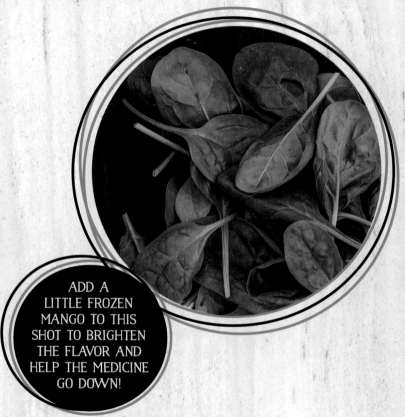

ADD A
LITTLE FROZEN
MANGO TO THIS
SHOT TO BRIGHTEN
THE FLAVOR AND
HELP THE MEDICINE
GO DOWN!

SHOOT IT

- PUT THE SPINACH, ALOE VERA, LIME JUICE, AND
  SPIRULINA POWDER INTO A BLENDER.

- POUR IN THE WATER AND BLEND UNTIL SMOOTH.
  SERVE IMMEDIATELY.

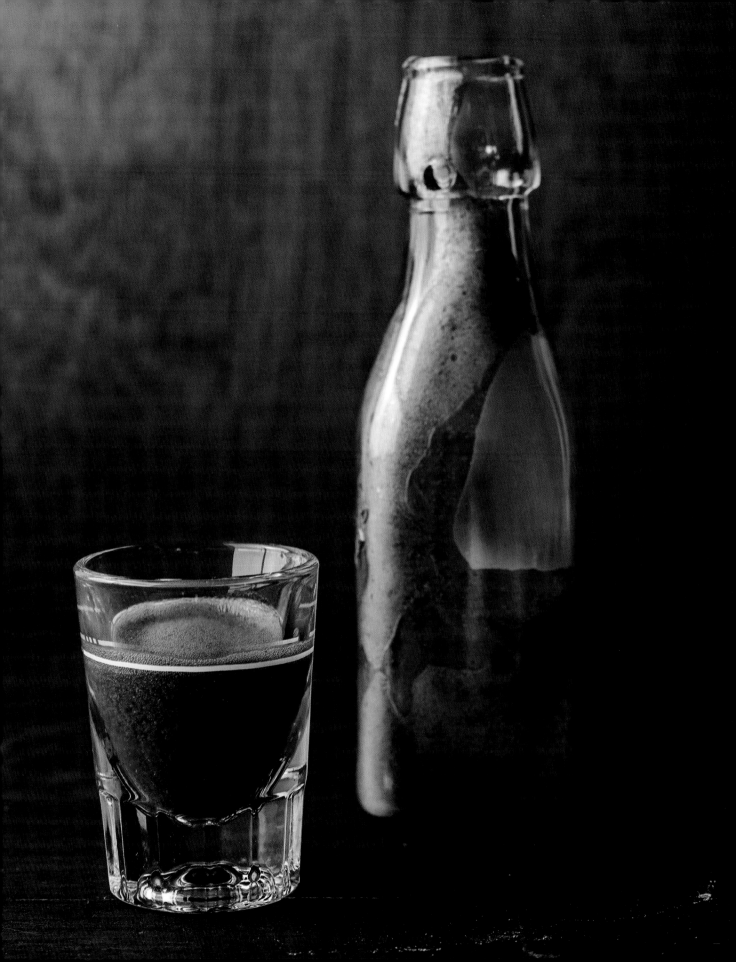

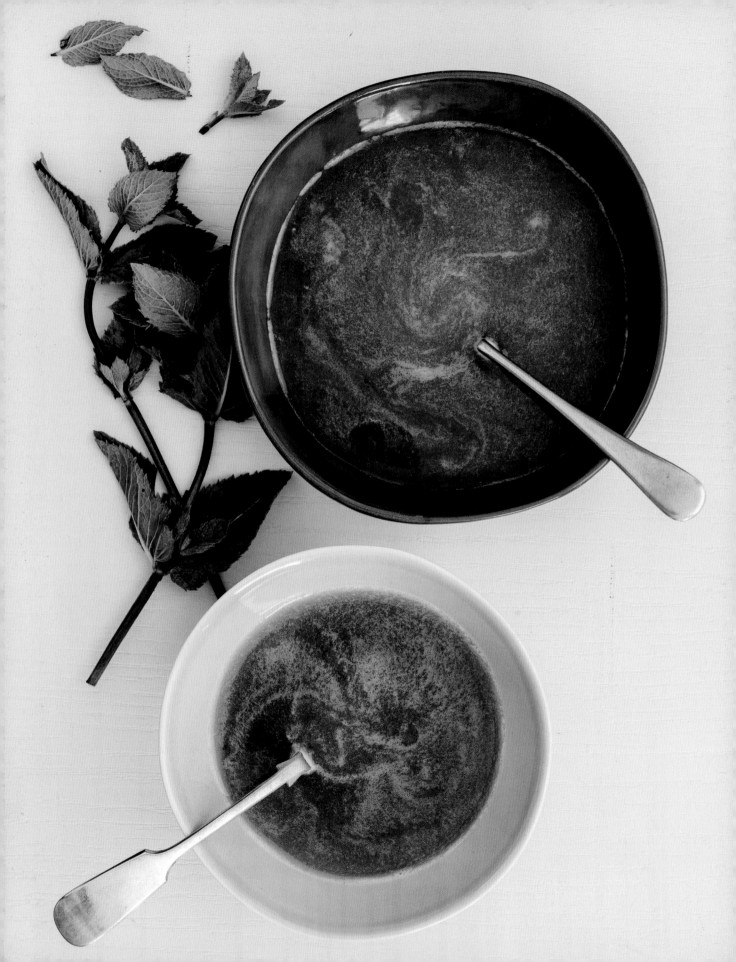

MELON BREEZE SOUP

UNLIKE WINTER SOUPS, WHICH WARM YOUR INSIDES, THIS SOUP WILL COOL YOU DOWN— PERFECT FOR A SUMMER APPETIZER OR AS PART OF YOUR LUNCH.

SERVES 1

Ingredients

½ LARGE GREEN MELON, PEELED AND SEEDED

1 CUCUMBER

¼ CUP CHOPPED FRESH MINT, PLUS A SPRIG TO GARNISH

1 cup chilled coconut water

MAKE THIS SOUP THE NIGHT BEFORE TO TAKE WITH YOU FOR LUNCH. IT WILL LOSE ITS VIBRANT COLOR SLIGHTLY AND SEPARATE, SO SHAKE IT JUST BEFORE SERVING.

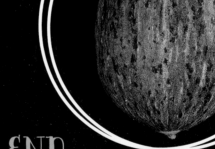

READY, STEADY ... BLEND

- CHOP THE MELON AND CUCUMBER AND PUT INTO A BLENDER.

- ADD THE MINT, POUR IN THE COCONUT WATER, AND BLEND UNTIL SMOOTH AND CREAMY.

- SERVE IMMEDIATELY OR CHILL IN THE REFRIGERATOR AND STIR JUST BEFORE SERVING. GARNISH WITH A SPRIG OF MINT.

INDEX

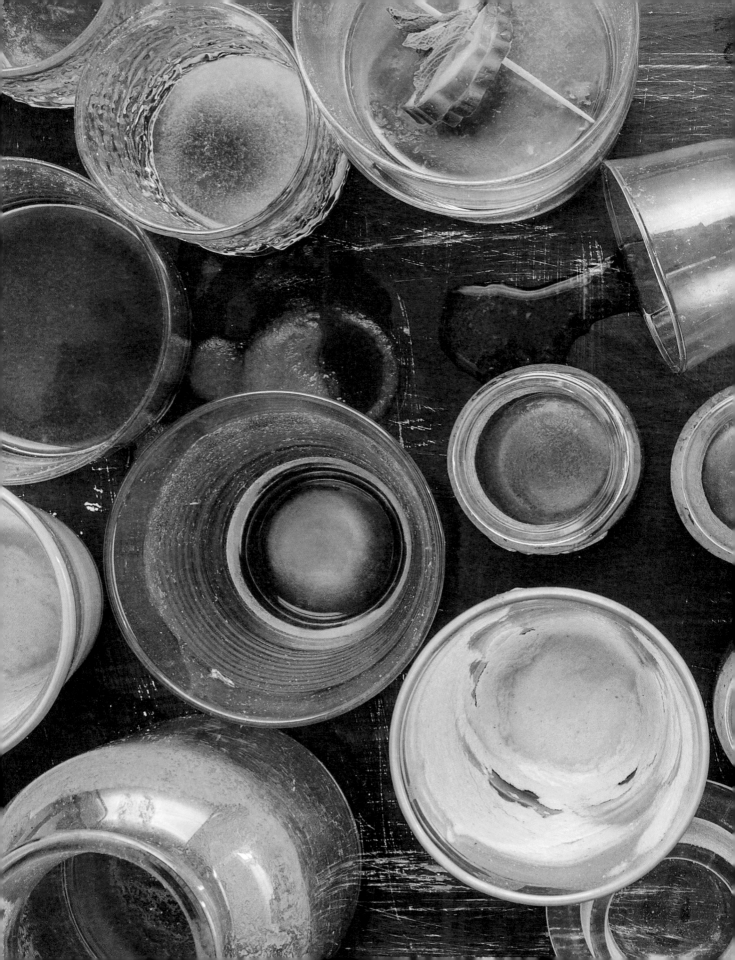